ESSENTIAL SKILLS IN FAMILY THERAPY

THE GUILFORD FAMILY THERAPY SERIES
Michael P. Nichols, Series Editor

Recent Volumes

Essential Skills in Family Therapy:
From the First Interview to Termination
JoEllen Patterson, Lee Williams, Claudia Grauf-Grounds, and Larry Chamow

Case Studies in Couple and Family Therapy: Systemic
and Cognitive Perspectives
Frank M. Dattilio, Editor

Working with Relationship Triangles:
The One-Two-Three of Psychotherapy
Philip J. Guerin, Jr., Thomas F. Fogarty, Leo F. Fay, and Judith Gilbert Kautto

Power and Compassion: Working with
Difficult Adolescents and Abused Parents
Jerome A. Price

If Problems Talked: Narrative Therapy in Action
Jeffrey L. Zimmerman and Victoria C. Dickerson

Narrative Solutions in Brief Therapy
Joseph B. Eron and Thomas W. Lund

Doing Family Therapy: Craft and Creativity in
Clinical Practice
Robert Taibbi

Learning and Teaching Therapy
Jay Haley

Treating People in Families:
An Integrative Framework
William C. Nichols

The Reflecting Team in Action:
Collaborative Practice in Family Therapy
Steven Friedman, Editor

Rewriting Family Scripts: Improvisation and
Systems Change
John Byng-Hall

ESSENTIAL SKILLS IN FAMILY THERAPY

From the First Interview to Termination

JOELLEN PATTERSON
LEE WILLIAMS
CLAUDIA GRAUF-GROUNDS
LARRY CHAMOW

Foreword by Douglas H. Sprenkle

THE GUILFORD PRESS
New York   London

© 1998 The Guilford Press
A Division of Guilford Publications, Inc.
72 Spring Street, New York, NY 10012
http://www.guilford.com

Printed in the United States of America

This book is printed on acid-free paper.

Last digit is print number: 9 8 7 6 5 4

Library of Congress Cataloging-in-Publication Data

Essential skills in family therapy: from the first interview to
termination / JoEllen Patterson . . . [et al.].
    p. cm. — (Guilford family therapy series)
Includes bibliographical references and index.
ISBN 1–57230–307–7 (hbk. : alk. paper)
    1. Family psychotherapy. 2. Family psychotherapy—Practice.
I. Patterson, JoEllen. II. Series.
RC488.5.P72 1998
616.89'156—DC21   97–41754
                                                              CIP

This book is dedicated to
George Sargent, PhD,
a friend, mentor, and colleague

Acknowledgments

This book is a joint effort of the authors but would never have come to fruition without the help of other colleagues. First we want to thank Leita McIntosh-Koontz, MA whose unmatched editorial skills kept this book on track; we are convinced it would never have been finished without her gentle persuasion to keep working at it. We also want to thank our dean, Ed DeRoche, PhD, who has supported the growth of the marriage and family therapy program at the University of San Diego (USD) since its creation 10 years ago. He has also supported us individually by providing financial resources and personal support. This book and the marriage and family therapy program would not have happened without him.

Our colleagues at USD, Rich Bischoff, Christie Turner, Moises Baron, Mel Mackler, and others, provide an intellectually and personally challenging atmosphere for work and study. Our students challenge us to keep finding new ways to teach family therapy. Finally, we are most grateful to our own families and the inspiration they provide for our work.

Foreword

As the immediate past editor of the *Journal of Marital and Family Therapy*, I was aware that some of the most interesting, innovative, and helpful articles on marriage and family therapy training were being written by faculty associated with the marital and family therapy (MFT) program at the University of San Diego. Therefore, I was not surprised when some members of this same group produced this enlightening book, specifically written for beginning family therapists.

I believe that this volume fills a significant gap in the literature where there is a need for an up-to-date and comprehensive "how to" manual that specifically addresses beginners' anxieties and limited knowledge regarding the "nuts and bolts" of treatment; as well as the administrative and political issues that surround MFT treatment at the approach of the next century.

Heretofore, the books we have given beginning therapists were typically of two types. Either we asked them to read the treatment models of the "masters," or we gave them one of the several MFT textbooks now available. Although the former are often inspiring, they often advocate a model that is not a good "match" for the student, create a "one-size-(model)-fits-all" mentality that does not square with the realities of practice, and frequently offer unrealistic case examples that showcase the masters' successes with difficult cases (and typically ignore their failures). They don't address the beginners' anxieties and may even enhance anxiety when the neophyte begins the often impossible translation of the master's ideas and techniques into his/her own practice. These textbooks do an excellent job of summarizing the history of the discipline and the broad strokes of MFT theories. However, they typically give short shrift to what one actually does before, during, and after sessions. This job of "translation" is typically left to supervisors, in-service training, and the trial-and-error learning that occurs in practica and internships.

While the authors of this book acknowledge that the core competencies of therapy cannot be taught didactically, they certainly offer the beginning therapist the best road map to acquiring these skills that I have ever seen. This volume will also be useful to experienced individual therapists who are beginning to make the transition to seeing families. Parts of the book, for example, the authors' excellent summaries of the clinical implications of recent research on the systemic treatment of disorders like depression, manic depressive illness, and anxiety disorders, can also be instructive to seasoned clinicians. I feel confident that many skilled family therapy trainers will use this manual as a resource for teaching beginners skills such as writing treatment plans, assessing for suicidality, violence, substance abuse, and duty-to-warn issues; and learning the basics about mental illness, psychopharmacology, and referral.

One main strength of *Essential Skills in Family Therapy* is its comprehensiveness. From a chapter discussing the initial apprehensions a novice has before seeing his/her first client to a strong chapter on the typically underplayed theme of termination, this book leaves few issues undiscussed. Although the major emphasis is on the "how to's" of practice, there is also a strong "self-of-the-therapist" subtheme in most chapters. I think this is especially important in a book geared to beginners since they frequently lack confidence (or occasionally may be too confident), wonder about their credibility, and frequently feel overwhelmed. The clarity with which the book is written, gearing the illustrations to beginners, and the step-by-step approach to the topics discussed makes the complexity of the therapeutic enterprise much less formidable to the reader.

Closely related, the book takes a "common factors" approach to therapeutic efficacy in that it stresses that there is precious little evidence for the differential effect of the various family therapy theoretical treatment models that we tend to hold so dear. Rather, the authors correctly note that the only solid research evidence we have is for the potency of a strong therapeutic relationship—a fact often ignored even by senior MFT educators and trainers (Sprenkle, Blow, and Dickey, in press). This is comforting to novices since they often feel more confident about joining and building bonds with clients than they do about implementing theory-driven techniques. The book does not ignore such techniques but rather demonstrates how a trainee can draw upon several different models (either singly or in combination) to formulate treatment plans/goals and related interventions. The authors wisely note that all helpful family therapies have an impact, although in differing degrees, on behaviors, cognitions, and emotions, and that none of the classic models has a monopoly on truth.

Students are urged to draw upon those models that make most sense to them, and with which they are comfortable, but also to formulate goals in collaboration with clients and to make sure that the tasks/interventions they use are credible to their clients.

I also appreciate the book's having a clear bio–psycho–social orientation. The authors align with Shields, McDaniel, and Wynne's (1994) concern that family therapy not become "marginalized" and treat MFT as a mental health discipline in dialogue with other disciplines. The authors are quite frank that MFT is not a "cure-all" and delineate the types of problems and circumstances calling for the services of other professionals. While some family therapy purists will object to the attention given to DSM-IV diagnoses and what to do when family members have mental illnesses, I think that it is imperative for beginning family therapists to learn this information if they are to practice in the current environment, whether or not they accept the epistemology and underlying assumptions of the mental health establishment.

The book does not shy away from controversy and presents a balanced treatment of issues ranging from the "false memory" debate, to handling secrets in therapy, to the realities of managed care. Case illustrations, used throughout, are realistic and portray (refreshingly) failures as well as successes. The administrative issues related to treatment—like informed consent, releases, videotaping, fee collection, and record keeping are not only explained but illustrative forms, including an intake form, a general assessment plan, suicide evaluations, treatment plans, a list of interventive questions, and a self-assessment when the therapist gets "stuck," are interspersed throughout the text.

In the last analysis, this book will make the reader more self-reflexive about what he or she is doing. I have long believed that family therapy trainers need to teach their trainers to "self-supervise," which is the meta-goal toward which this book seems to be pointing. Reading and digesting this book may help the novice to feel like he/she is carrying with him/her a wise and compassionate supervisor. As with the person who mentored me, this book speaks with clinical wisdom, clarity, gentleness, sensitivity, and flexibility, and I believe it will empower beginning therapists to do their best work. I am sure we will use this book at Purdue University and feel confident it will have a wide audience throughout the MFT landscape. The authors are all to be commended for producing what will be the benchmark volume for beginning therapists for many years to come.

DOUGLAS H. SPRENKLE, PHD
Professor of Marriage and Family Therapy,
Purdue University

REFERENCES

Shields, C., Wynne, L., McDaniel, S., & Gawinski, B. (1994). The marginalization of family therapy: A historical and continuing problem. *Journal of Marital and Family Therapy, 20,* 117–138.

Sprenkle, D., Blow, A., & Dickey, M. (in press). Common factors and other non model-driven technique variables in marriage and family therapy. In M. A. Hubbell, B. L. Duncan, & S. Miller (Eds.), *The heart and soul of change: Common factors in effective psychotherapy, medicine, and human services.* Washington, DC: American Psychological Association.

Contents

1

The Beginning Family Therapist: Taking on the Challenge

Tom is handed the intake paperwork for his first client at his new practicum site. Both excited and anxious, he scans the information. In the section on "primary reason for coming to therapy" the client has written "need ways to cope with my husband's drinking and his hitting the children." Tom grows more apprehensive as he wonders where to start. Should he simply listen to the woman's story as it unfolds? Or should he take a more direct approach and immediately assess for a substance abuse problem? Still another focus is the indication of child abuse. Perhaps this very serious matter takes precedence over every other issue.

Sally reviews today's back-to-back schedule and wonders if she will make it through the day. After learning yesterday that her father has cancer and is likely to die within the year, she tossed and turned all night. Exhausted but wanting to do a good job with her clients, she begins thinking about her first client family that day. The Joneses have an 8-year-old son with a multitude of problems: leukemia and attention-deficit/hyperactivity disorder, to name two. He has been referred by the family's physician "to develop coping skills." For a fleeting moment, Sally wonders if the pain she feels about her father will affect her therapy today, but she does not have much time to reflect on this question because her first session starts in 5 minutes.

Ann winces as she recalls her group supervision session yesterday. She had thought the videotaped session of her work with Mrs. Thomas showed what excellent joining skills she had. It would be clear to her supervisor and her fellow students that Mrs. Thomas liked therapy and took Ann's suggestions very seriously. But instead of focusing on the therapist–client rapport, the group had overwhelmed Ann with assessment questions she had not even considered. How was Mrs. Thomas's divorce connected to her depression? Did Ann think her late-night alcohol use reflected a substance abuse problem? Were Mrs. Thomas's children being neglected because she had little energy or time for parenting? What should Ann's level of involvement be in "helping" Mrs. Thomas find a job? Ann wondered if she had the necessary qualities to even be the therapist when she had so clearly missed important assessment questions for her client.

Most beginning therapists experience a host of anxious feelings when they start clinical work. They are aware of their inadequacies more than their strengths, and need help to learn how to acquire the skills, knowledge, and sense of competency necessary to do good clinical work.

Many therapists complete the didactic part of their training with a sense of mastery and competence. After all, by the time they enter graduate school, the life of a student is very familiar, and they are accustomed to academic achievement in their course work. Academic accomplishments, however, do not necessarily translate into therapeutic competence. Indeed, Figley and Nelson (1989) have pointed out that most of the core competencies of therapists are qualities that cannot be taught in a traditional didactic manner. Faculty and students are left wondering how best to impart and acquire, respectively, the skills basic to clinical work.

The gap between academic work and the implementation of techniques or the application of theories in clinical sessions can seem huge. After a year of intense academic instruction, students often begin their clinical work with unstated questions:

"What am I supposed to say to the client?"

"How do I handle situation X?"

"What should happen after I complete the intake form?"

"Can clients tell I'm new at this and feeling completely inadequate and overwhelmed?"

"How do I keep all the information from the session clear and how do I know what is most important?"

"If I don't use a powerful intervention or technique during the first couple of sessions, am I a failure?"

"I know I should have a theory for this case but I just don't understand how to apply information from my theories class to this acting-out adolescent and her hostile mother."

"How will I know if the clients actually get better?"

What students need is a way to develop their skills as therapists as they begin their clinical work. This book provides practical, "how to" guidelines on essential therapeutic skills from thorough assessment to careful treatment planning, from the nuts and bolts of specific interventions to the nuances of establishing therapeutic relationships and troubleshooting when treatment gets "stuck."

Reflecting the trend toward integrative approaches in family therapy, mental health, and the medical field, we stress a biopsychosocial view of assessment and treatment. This approach is designed to meet the changing demands of mental health care provision, and it means that beginning family therapists will need to acquire new skills and hone traditional ones. The concrete guidelines in this book address these issues. For example, therapists are increasingly required to assess, diagnose, and treat clients in a more expedient manner. The existence of new research on the efficacy of specific treatments for specific problems means that therapists must know the literature on a certain problem or diagnosis. Dubbed "differential therapeutics" and the "specificity question" by diverse professionals, the issue of treatment fit was judged by Piercy and Sprenkle (1990) to be fundamental to therapy in this decade. In their review of the previous decade of family therapy research, these authors highlight the question of "what treatment works best for what problem under what set of circumstances" (p. 1120).

The ability to integrate family therapy theory and interventions with individual diagnosis and treatment will be especially valuable as therapists begin their careers. While family therapy offers a unique and important perspective in clinical work, much of what goes on in treatment shares common assumptions with all therapies. Certain clinical skills—assessing for suicide risk or substance abuse, making an effective referral—are intrinsic to any good therapy. This book goes beyond the boundaries of traditional family therapy to be as inclusive as possible of essential clinical skills.

Frequently, beginning family therapy students make treatment decisions based on their supervisors' favorite theoretical orientation or the specific theoretical approach predominant in their clinic. We believe that assessing the appropriateness of a family therapy treatment for a specific problem is an essential clinical skill. It is important to be able to recognize when a problem is outside the scope of a family therapist's practice (or skill level) and could best be treated by another mental health professional or in tandem with another health care professional.

Indeed, research on biological etiologies of mental illness and psychopharmacology suggests that therapists must be conversant with more than "talk therapies." A growing focus on treatment teams and multidisciplinary treatment approaches means that therapists must increasingly attend to the biological component of the biopsychosocial model and learn to collaborate with other health care professionals. A knowledge base in medication management and the ability to consult with physicians is one aspect of this new approach.

In addition, strong demands for quality assurance, timeliness, and cost-effectiveness are being placed on therapists by managed care companies. The movement toward quality assurance panels and set-treatment protocols in managed care suggests that students must learn the state of the art treatment for a given problem. Consideration of these changes underlie many of the approaches and practices discussed in this book, fitting with our view that current clinical issues go beyond the beginning therapist's need to translate theory into practice. Thus, while family interaction remains a focus of attention herein, our goal is to prepare beginning therapists to integrate information and skills in order to best meet the needs of diverse client families.

While the bulk of this book discusses specific processes and skills that are important throughout the therapeutic journey, we devote the first chapter to that most basic of concerns for the beginning therapist—understanding and managing beginners' jitters.

GETTING STARTED

"It was my first session with a client and my heart was racing. I had no idea what to do with this family, and I wasn't really sure if they knew why they were all there. I was talking with the mother, who requested the appointment, to find out how much the other family members knew about why they came in when I realized that I didn't really like this lady. . . ."

This story, shared by a practicum student, encompasses two essential and pressing issues shared by most beginning therapists. One revolves around the question "What to do?" and the other involves managing one's own feelings and reactions to diverse clients and clinical situations.

Learning the art and science of doing therapy is a challenging task, particularly when first seeing clients. Many beginning therapists have periodic feelings of inadequacy and insecurity about their clinical abilities. Some may fear that they will directly harm their clients or cause their condition to deteriorate because of clinical mistakes. Others fear that they will not be able to help their clients because of their inexperience. A few doubt their talent and ability as therapists to the extent that they seriously question whether or not to remain in the field.

Therapists and supervisors alike need to see confidence issues from a developmental perspective. Given their lack of clinical experience, it is only natural that beginning therapists question their competence. In fact, as supervisors, we worry more about beginning therapists who seem extremely confident in their abilities. This feeling of confidence is incongruent with the complexity and difficulty of learning to do therapy well.

MANAGING ANXIETY
AND ISSUES OF CONFIDENCE

How does the beginning therapist deal with a lack of confidence, or with feeling overwhelmed and anxious? First, therapists must recognize that these feelings are completely normal. Although the intensity of the feelings and the way of coping will vary from therapist to therapist, every beginning therapist struggles to some degree with these feelings. Therapists who do not acknowledge this often get trapped in a vicious circle. They interpret feelings of being overwhelmed as a possible sign that they are not cut out to be therapists, which only serves to fuel their anxiety.

Second, beginning therapists need to share these experiences with other therapists and supervisors. Sharing feelings of anxiety or lack of confidence can help to normalize the experience. Unfortunately, it is fear of being incompetent or a failure that prevents beginning therapists from sharing their struggles with others. When a therapist does take the risk and shares his or her fears with peers, others generally disclose the same worries. This in turn helps the beginning therapist to accept that these struggles are developmentally appropriate rather than a sign of being unsuited for the profession.

Third, distorted cognitions or beliefs may contribute to a therapist's fears or struggles with confidence. These can be addressed using cognitive restructuring. The first step is for the therapist to identify cognitions or beliefs about the ability to do therapy effectively. For example, some beginners have questioned the ethicality of treating difficult clients (or any client at all!) when more experienced therapists are available. When distortions are identified, perhaps with a supervisor's help, they can be "replaced" with more constructive thoughts that benefit coping and decrease anxiety. Recalling that such seasoned clinicians as Salvador Minuchin and Virginia Satir were once beginners can help. A good battery of constructive thoughts and images goes a long way toward soothing beginners' jitters.

Fourth, it is crucial to realize that the therapist–client relationship is inherently therapeutic. A therapist doesn't need to *do* something to be experienced positively by clients. This is very reassuring to most beginning therapists because they generally have confidence in their relational skills. When beginning therapists are instructed as to the importance of joining and empathically listening to their clients, most therapists are relieved, feeling "I can do that!"

Finally, beginning therapists need to recognize that their early experiences in seeing clients often involve a steep learning curve, like any other new job. You will be less anxious doing an intake with a family if you have one or two intakes "under your belt." It takes time, however, to gain enough experience before many situations become familiar.

Many beginning therapists wonder at what point they will stop struggling with issues of confidence. Experienced clinicians indicated that after 5 to 7 years (or about 5,000 to 7,000 hours) of clinical experience, they had encountered most clinical issues or problems several times before. As a result, they felt very secure or confident in their abilities as therapists.

Fortunately, therapists don't need to complete 5,000 to 7,000 hours of work to see a notable improvement in their confidence. The intense feelings of anxiety and being overwhelmed that are common in the very beginning generally subside after a month or so of seeing clients. Beginning therapists also become less fearful that they will do something to harm their clients, although they continue to struggle with feelings of being ineffective or unhelpful.

Obtaining 500 to 700 hours appears to be another significant turning point in the growth of therapist confidence. At this level of experience, beginning therapists generally report greater confidence in conceptualizing cases. They often report knowing what needs to be changed, but are unsure of how to intervene to bring that change about.

Most therapists will have confidence in their overall abilities by the time they have had 1,000 to 1,500 hours of clinical experience. At this point, they are better at conceptualizing cases and have also developed a repertoire of effective interventions. Of course, therapists can still experience periodic doubts about their abilities, particularly when struggling with difficult cases or issues. Issues of confidence may also reemerge if therapists start working with new and unfamiliar populations. However, most therapists at this stage are not plagued by doubts about their clinical ability.

STAGES OF THERAPIST DEVELOPMENT

McCollum (1990) notes that therapists trained in individual therapy generally go through three stages of development when learning to do family therapy. In the first stage, they focus on acquiring the skills necessary to work with families. In the second stage, they learn to apply systemic theory to their clinical work, and in the third, "self of the therapist" stage, they focus on more personal issues in relationship to their clinical work, such as exploring how their family of origin experiences affect their work with families.

Although McCollum's observations were based on teaching experienced therapists to do family therapy, these stages also apply to individuals learning family therapy without prior clinical experience. In essence, the initial skills stage is characterized by therapists trying to figure out what to do with clients. This focus then shifts in the theory stage to how to think. In the final stage, the therapist focuses on the use of self in being with a family.

Although each stage has a particular emphasis, all three may overlap from time to time. While developmental stages are differentiated by time and experience, other factors can bring any or all of their foci to the fore— particular client families and clinical issues, the emphasis of a certain supervisor or training program, and the abiding interests of the therapist, among others.

Stage One: Learning Essential Skills

Before therapists start their clinical work, they often experience a mixture of feelings. Most report an excitement at finally beginning to "do" therapy, and some even express impatience to see clients. They are eager to apply what they have learned in their classes by working with people in therapy. But the predominant emotion that most therapists report before seeing their first client is significant anxiety.

It is natural for therapists to have these worries before they see their first client and even after they begin to work. Beginning therapists report feeling overwhelmed by the experience. Many report going home after seeing clients and crying, while others report that the stress results in headaches, difficulty sleeping, stomachaches, or changes in appetite.

This early stage is a time for beginners to learn and practice basic skills. Learning to relax and be present in the therapy room with first clients is a good place to start. A solid assessment and effective treatment hinge on the therapist's ability to listen and attend to the client's story, and to show the client that he or she is understood. Beginners can learn to replace their anxiety about "doing something" with relaxed curiosity and empathy. This approach leads to useful questions and inquiries, which is where therapy begins.

Stage Two: Learning to Conceptualize Cases

Beginning therapists soon recognize that the therapeutic relationship is a necessary but not always sufficient ingredient for change. They no longer are content simply to be with their clients; they realize that some clients need concrete ideas or suggestions for change. At the same time, therapists also become aware that to be effective, interventions must be rooted in a clear understanding of family dynamics. As a result, therapists soon move into a second stage, where emphasis is placed on conceptualizing what is happening in their cases.

Learning to conceptualize cases can be difficult and frustrating. In this stage, therapists frequently struggle with issues such as the following:

> "How do I know what is the most important information to attend to in a case?"
>
> "My clients keep coming in with a different problem each week. How do I figure out what to focus on?"
>
> "I know I should have theory for this case, but I'm not sure what theory would 'work' here."
>
> "I thought I knew what we should be working on last week, but now I'm confused again."
>
> "I know I should be focusing on the process, but I feel like I'm stuck in the content."

Typically, beginning therapists are able to develop good insights and hypotheses, but will have difficulty connecting these pieces together into a coherent picture or treatment plan. Gradually, there will be moments of clarity wherein the pieces fit together. With the passage of time, these moments begin to last longer than the periods of haze and confusion.

Early in the second stage, many therapists find it helpful to adopt a particular theoretical orientation for conceptualizing cases (McCollum, 1990). As they gain intensive experience with one theoretical framework, they begin to recognize its limitations and may try others. As therapists explore different theories, they eventually develop their own framework, integrating the best parts of the different orientations that they have adopted.

Stage Three: The Therapist-as-Self

As therapists become more skilled at and comfortable with conceptualizing cases, they shift more of their focus to looking at themselves in therapy. There is a growing recognition that the self of the therapist can greatly influence therapy, and beginning family therapists gradually become more interested in identifying their unique contributions to the therapeutic encounter.

During this stage, therapists will often explore how the therapist-as-self is both an asset and liability in therapy. Many of our personal experiences can become catalysts for new ideas and understanding in therapeutic work. For example, a therapist who has been able to successfully develop an adult-to-adult relationship with his or her parents may use that personal experience in working with clients who are struggling with issues of differentiation. Specific life experiences—trauma, parenthood, separation, illness—may all come into play in a way that benefits therapeutic work.

However, therapists' unresolved issues or "growth areas" can become impediments in therapy. Therefore, some therapists choose to explore their personal issues more closely at this stage, often by seeking therapy for themselves. The growth and insight derived from working on these issues can provide the perspective necessary to make constructive use of life experiences in therapy.

OBSESSING ABOUT CLINICAL WORK

Many beginning therapists report that they cannot stop thinking about therapy or their clients. In fact, thinking about clients seems to fill every waking moment and even many nonwaking moments. It is not unusual for beginning therapists to report having dreams about their clients or doing therapy.

Learning to do anything new, particularly something as challenging as therapy, can easily consume much of one's time, thoughts, and energy. Furthermore, most people who choose therapy as a profession have a deep compassion and concern for people. It is often difficult not to think about clients, particularly when they are in considerable pain or distress.

Thinking (or even obsessing) about clients is something that tends to subside with time and experience. Most experienced therapists report thinking very little about their clients outside the therapy hour. One reason for this change is that the therapist gradually gains a greater sense of clinical mastery by virtue of experience. In addition, therapists learn to balance objectivity and emotional involvement with clients. In a sense, therapists learn how to construct an emotional boundary. If the boundary becomes too diffuse, the therapist may be overwhelmed and inducted into the family system. If it is too rigid, he or she may lack the empathy necessary to adequately understand the issues and join with the family. The former problem is characteristic of beginning therapists, who, with time, learn to better regulate this boundary.

CONCLUSION

Building confidence and competence in one's clinical work is part of the larger process of learning to do good therapy. The greatest task for a beginning family therapist lies in developing a clear understanding of clinical issues and an ability to apply therapeutic skills, to which we devote the remainder of this book.

Chapters 2–6 follow the usual time sequence of therapy—from initial contact with clients, to comprehensive assessment, to treatment planning and intervention. Mental health skills needed by all therapists are intertwined with family therapy knowledge. Our goal here is to provide beginning therapists with the tools for thinking about clinical issues, rather than merely applying an approach propounded by their instructors.

Chapters 7–9 deal with specific clinical situations based on presenting problems and the nature of client families. We examine major issues and approaches for working with children and adolescents, couples, and families that are struggling with serious mental illness.

Chapter 10 highlights some common obstacles all therapists encounter, and provides concrete ideas on how to get unstuck when treatment is not progressing. Chapter 11 focuses on an often overlooked part of therapy—termination. In Chapter 12, we conclude the book by examining the implications of health care reform on our work as family therapists. Recognizing that changes in health care will create the context, limits, and parameters in which therapists practice, we make a few brief suggestions on preparing for the future.

2

Before the Initial Interview

$\mathbf{M}$rs. Escutia's voice quivers nervously over the phone line at a community counseling clinic, "I must speak to a counselor . . . please!" she exclaims. "My grandson is in trouble, he needs help. I don't know what to do any more. I'm afraid he could. . . ." The clinic intake worker jots down a few notes and quickly calls up one of the clinic's family therapy interns. "I've got a woman on the phone whose grandson just killed a hamster with a shovel," the intake worker says. "Can you take her?" For a brief moment, the new client and the new intern share a silent space filled with questions and anxieties. The first contact is about to take place, and it can easily make or break a future collaboration where healing work can be done.

DEALING WITH FAMILIES' EXPECTATIONS
AND ANXIETIES ABOUT THERAPY

Were it possible to stop action, as we have done in the preceding case material, we would capture a glimpse of one of the most critical periods of the therapeutic experience—before therapy ever begins. It is during this fragile period that prospective clients decide if they want to risk going to therapy. While clients with previous positive therapy experiences may reinitiate treatment with a hopeful attitude, others have ambivalent hopes, expectations, and fears about beginning therapy.

Consider Mrs. Escutia. In her family, problems have traditionally been handled by husbands and wives, aunts and uncles, grandparents, long-time friends, and others who are close to the family hearth. Her anxiety

11

about calling in "professional" help is matched only by her concern for her grandson, whose violent temper has pushed the entire family past its limits. With no previous experience in therapy, she wonders what a stranger in this clinic could possibly do to help—after all, everything has been tried! Will this counselor believe her? How should she present this terrible dilemma? Will anyone out there really care? Does seeking help mean she has failed?

It is not uncommon for families to be at their wit's end when they finally decide to seek treatment or are otherwise referred and call for an appointment. Chances are they're worn out, fed up, and feeling hopeless. Further, individual family members may differ remarkably in their attitudes, expectations, and motivations regarding a try at therapy. They may have both overt and covert reasons for coming to therapy, and rarely are the family members' reasons the same. Uncovering much of this information may not occur until the first interview or even beyond, but it is a good idea to keep the following questions in mind right from the first contact:

"What are the clients' expectations about therapy?"
"What are their anxieties about coming to therapy?"
"What motivates them to come to therapy, and who is the referral source?"
"Why do they want to come to therapy now?"

If the therapist isn't aware of the often hidden issues related to clients' motivation, expectations, and anxieties, he or she may inadvertently respond in a manner that causes clients to decide that therapy is not worth the risk, or, conversely, that leads to accepting clients who might be better served elsewhere. For example, beginning therapists may find themselves drawn into legal cases that involve divorce, custody, adoption, or numerous other types of litigation. Family therapists are seldom trained in the specifics of mediation or custody evaluation, and, for most of us, it is best to decline doing therapy in such situations.

Even in cases where therapy is clearly indicated and doesn't involve potential legal tangles, family members' reasons for starting treatment and levels of motivation are important to assess. In individual work, these issues may be less salient because rarely do individuals come to therapy without wanting to be there. Conjoint treatment presents a different picture. For example, in couple therapy there is often one person who is more motivated to come to therapy or at least views therapy as an effective method for dealing with relationship problems. The partner may be resistant to treatment, have other preferred solutions for addressing marital issues, or be willing to come to therapy only if it is framed as a way to "help my partner" or "save the marriage."

With families, reasons and motivations for therapy vary further. Perhaps one powerful family member is coercing others to attend. Perhaps the safety of a "neutral" therapist and a scheduled weekly hour is necessary for a family to talk together about personal and significant issues. In addition, referral sources and previous treatment are absolutely crucial to consider when gauging family members' diverse responses to seeing a therapist. Court-ordered treatment may indicate a potentially resistant or reluctant client, though this is by no means the rule. Referrals by school counselors, ministers, physicians, or family friends will likely influence how families first approach treatment. For example, family members may not agree with a school counselor's view of "the problem" and as a result have little investment in seeking therapy. On the other hand, such a referral from a perceived "professional" may be just the validation the family needs to actively seek help. Similarly, the nature of previous contacts with other agencies or individuals may predispose a family to have enormous expectations for therapy, or none at all. Since these rarely articulated expectations and anxieties will alter how a therapist approaches treatment with a new family, it is essential to get a "feel" for them from the outset.

Clients like Mrs. Escutia will have as many questions swirling about as the therapist does when the first contact is made. Topping the list may be concerns about the therapist's ability to truly understand and care, and questions about whether he or she can actually help. Clients may find answers to these questions in how quickly their phone calls are returned or in their sense that the listener understands a brief explanation of the problem. The therapist's (or agency's) flexibility in responding to individual needs communicates answers to these questions. The degree of focus on charges and payments versus listening to the client may communicate that the client is not a priority—money is. If the client decides, via these early perceptions, that the therapist doesn't care or can't help, the initial session may never happen. On the other hand, an initial call that relays empathy and confidence can begin to create the foundation upon which a successful therapy can be built.

SUGGESTIONS FOR INITIAL CONTACT WITH THE CLIENT

Keeping in mind the myriad expectations, anxieties, and questions of potential clients, therapists can be guided through the first-time telephone conversation by using a number of pragmatic suggestions for handling initial contacts:

1. *Listen and reflect to the client what you hear.* Simply by listening and briefly reflecting what is said, you can help the prospective client feel

he has been heard. Effective listening can be done in 5 minutes and the client can hang up with a new sense of hope about resolving the problem.

2. *Assess if this is a crisis situation.* The initial phone call may indicate a need for immediate crisis intervention, hospitalization, removal of family members from the home, and/or involvement of other agencies such as police or child protective services. Therapists should be knowledgeable about the clinic's or agency's protocol for handling crises, and of community or state laws that may apply (e.g., child abuse reporting laws).

3. *Consider scope-of-practice issues.* Do you have the knowledge and experience to diagnose and treat the presenting problem? Some agencies carefully screen the clients that beginning therapists treat. For example, a problem that is primarily biomedical, one that involves suicide risk or serious drug and alcohol use, or a purely individualized problem (such as a phobia) may not be within the scope of practice for a marriage and family therapist. You can begin clarifying your strengths and limits immediately.

4. *Respond as promptly as possible.* Return phone calls, set up the initial session, and complete an assessment as quickly as you can. These behaviors indicate that you take the client's concerns seriously and are competent to respond to his or her needs. You create a sense of credibility and ensure the client that you can help early on.

5. *Consider why this particular family member made the initial contact and keep in mind that a sense of rapport with each individual in the family is important.* Therapists often make several mistakes around this issue. It is easy to be drawn to the most "psychologically minded" or powerful client and inadvertently ignore those who are likely part of the problem as well as part of the solution. Before the first session, the family member who made the phone call is in essence the family spokesperson. However, the therapist may want contact with other family members before the first session. The goal of additional phone contacts is to make sure every family member feels welcome and knows that their feelings and ideas matter to the therapist.

6. *Address the "business" of therapy as quickly and efficiently as possible while not detracting from the client's need to be heard.* Basic explanations about fees and payment, how to make appointments, and policies about keeping and canceling appointments are important. Transportation issues are relevant for many families, too. Do the clients have a car, or someone who can drive them to appointments? Must they navigate and pay for public transportation? Do they have directions to the clinic? What about family work and school schedules? Do they have childcare, if this is needed? Addressing such concerns up front can assist the therapist and family in avoiding no-shows and cancellations due to logistical problems that were never worked out. Issues such as informed consent and confidentiality may be dealt with on the telephone, or more

frequently through mailed information or forms provided at the clinic just before the first session. (Chapter 3 addresses these issues in detail.) Regardless of how this information is communicated, it is important to ensure that clients are clearly informed about what is expected of them and what they can expect from therapy.

7. *Limit the first contact by sticking to basic, relevant information and issues.* This is not the time to offer interventions, advice, or suggestions. Be prepared to direct the telephone interview. Prospective clients may be interested in lengthy venting of problems, in getting detailed information about your qualifications, methods, and philosophy, in obtaining an immediate diagnosis, or in any other manner of fact and opinion that, while valid, is best saved for a first meeting.

WHAT INFORMATION SHOULD BE OBTAINED?

Most agencies and therapists have an "intake" form that gathers basic information about the client during the initial contact. This information may be obtained by an "intake receptionist" or a therapist over the phone. Other possibilities include mailing the form to the client before the first session or having the client complete the form in the waiting room before the first session. Even when initial telephone contacts are time-limited and may not be as comprehensive as formal intake questionnaires, the call can still begin the processes of evaluation and joining by focusing on the following questions:

1. What is the problem and how does the client present it? Is this a crisis, a severe or moderate problem, a discrete situation, a chronic difficulty?
2. How has the family responded to the situation? How have they managed so far?
3. Has there been previous therapy?
4. Why is the family seeking treatment now?
5. What additional factors are influencing the situation (e.g., nature and frequency of various stressors—whether they are vocational, personal, physical, or otherwise)?

Figure 2.1 provides a sample intake form that reflects the information deemed most important by marriage and family therapists. The emphasis on specific information varies, depending on the training of the mental health professional. For example, most psychiatric intake forms focus on individual symptoms instead of relationships, whereas a child psychologist may include questions about a child's prenatal history and

Name: _____ Telephone: _____ Date of Birth: _____ Place of Birth: _____ Age: _____

Address: _____ Marital Status: _____ Religion: _____ Race: _____ Gender: _____

Place of Employment: _____ Length of Employment: _____

Last Place of Employment: _____ Length of Employment: _____

Address: _____ Supervisor: _____

Telephone: _____ Hours Worked: _____ Salary: _____

Education Completed: _____ Where: _____

Name(s) of Child/Children: _____ Date of Birth: _____ Age: _____ School Attended: _____

_____ _____ _____ _____

_____ _____ _____ _____

_____ _____ _____ _____

Have you (or spouse) ever been involved in therapy or any other type of counseling programs? ☐ Yes ☐ No

If yes, when?_____ Where? _____

Reasons: _____

Reasons for considering counseling at this time: _____

_____

Have you ever been referred to this agency? ☐ Yes ☐ No   If yes, by whom?_____

Reasons for the referral: _____

Are you in treatment with another counselor at this time? ☐ Yes ☐ No   If yes, with whom?_____

When?_____ How long?_____

Have you ever been hospitalized for any mental health reasons? ☐ Yes ☐ No If yes, when?_____

Where?_____ By whom?_____

Have you ever, or are you now being treated by any type of chemical dependency abuse? ☐ Yes ☐ No

If yes, when?_____ Where?_____

By whom?_____ Length of treatment?_____

Are you at the present time using any type of chemical substance? ☐ Yes ☐ No   If yes, please indicate what you are using (drugs and/or alcohol): _____

How frequently do you use these substances?_____

FIGURE 2.1. Sample intake form.

Are you presently under a physician's care for physical problems? ☐ Yes ☐ No

If yes, please list medication:_____

Name of family physician:_____ Telephone:_____

Address: _____

Have you ever been arrested and/or committed a crime? ☐ Yes ☐ No

If yes, when?_____ For what?_____

Outcome of situation: _____

What problems are you presently experiencing?_____

_____

What do you expect from therapy?_____

_____

Please list everyone in your family with whom you presently live:

_____   _____

_____   _____

_____   _____

_____   _____

Identify the primary problem(s) you are now experiencing:_____

_____

If need be, would other relatives be willing to come into therapy sessions? ☐ Yes ☐ No

If no, please indicate reason:_____

Person to contact in case of emergency:_____ Telephone:_____

Address:_____

_____   _____

Signature   Date

TO ALL CLIENTS:

If at any time you believe a concern arises in your treatment, please discuss it with your therapist.

Intake comments:

Preliminary treatment plans:

17

delivery. Regardless of the therapist's orientation, all intake forms should include a place for the client's brief description of the problem (in the client's own words), notes about previous treatments, and inquiries about current medications and medical problems. Whether this information is obtained during an initial phone contact or at the first session, it is crucial data that helps direct assessment and treatment.

WHO SHOULD COME TO THERAPY?

During the initial phone contact, the therapist needs to indicate that involvement of the family is critical. While most therapists are flexible enough not to insist that everyone involved be present at every session, an early message that therapy is usually a family affair lays the groundwork for involvement by members who may be perceived as peripheral to the problem. When the presenting problem clearly involves a relationship (sibling fights or parent–child standoffs), it is a useful general rule to get all the people in the relationship to come to therapy.

Beyond this basic principle, the following guidelines can help you determine, early on, the best possible format for new clients:

1. Ask the family who they want to come to therapy, and why.
2. Consider who is involved in the problem. Is the presenting problem directly related to current interactions in the family? If so, those involved should come to therapy.
3. Consider generational boundaries. Is it appropriate to have all age groups in therapy?
4. Even if the problem is primarily an individual one, would other family members' presence facilitate treatment or feel supportive to the individual?
5. Would other family members hinder the therapy and be potentially damaging?
6. What motivation and capacity does the family have to participate in a family format?
7. Be open to changing who comes for each session depending on the problem, but try to establish a relationship with all members.

Clients naturally have an opinion about who should come to therapy, and the reasons underlying such views should be considered and addressed. For example, sometimes a spouse will request individual therapy "because I'm the one causing the problems in the marriage." The therapist can point out that a relationship problem is involved and can recommend that both partners attend. Similarly, family members may consider the "identified patient" to be the only one who needs to come to therapy. Clearly, a direct relationship exists between treatment goals and who attends therapy. Therapy goals may be limited or broadened depending on the willingness of different family members to participate in therapy. As long as the relationship between participation and goals is clarified for the family when the terms of therapy are being established, there need not be any hard-and-fast rules about who comes to each session.

Doherty and Simmons (1995) note that family therapists are still most likely to see, in rank order, individuals, then couples, and then families. The public is just beginning to conceptualize problems as relational rather than intrapsychic, and probably still thinks of therapy as primarily an individual experience. Therapists may need to educate new clients about the benefits of conjoint treatment by emphasizing the power of relationships in influencing how people feel, think, and act. While there are times that individual therapy is appropriate (e.g., when victims of violence or incest must be separated from the perpetrator), family therapists generally focus on treating relationships by having all the players present.

INITIAL HYPOTHESIZING

After the initial contact, most therapists find themselves with enough basic information to begin forming a few hypotheses, which provide the therapist with areas to further pursue in the first interview. Questions should be designed to elicit data that will either support or invalidate the hypotheses.

In order to begin the process of clinical thinking the therapist needs to pay close attention to what is known and how that information might be useful. Too often we look quickly for underlying meanings of events before we have a working understanding of the presenting problem. It can be helpful to first summarize what information is available and then pick out the key issues. What is the client telling you that he or she thinks is important? Initially, the process of asking key questions will prove far more fruitful than making interpretations of the client's motives or behavior.

The process of developing hypotheses is an opportunity for creative thinking. Our guesses and speculations are based upon our previous experiences with similar cases, our knowledge about individual or family development, and our clinical hunches or intuitions. At this stage of the process, we are not looking for answers, but finding questions. Hypotheses relate to what may be happening or what events could have occurred. The therapist's position is not to presume to know, but assume to ask. The following example of a clinical situation shows how developing some hypotheses proves useful in beginning a clinical assessment.

A 9-year-old girl who has never really liked school suddenly refuses to go at all. She has become withdrawn and sullen. When asked why she doesn't want to go to school, she simply cries and refuses to answer. In order to develop some hypotheses about this case, it is first useful to note and summarize the key issues. The presenting problem is the child's refusal to go to school. Her response to being asked about the problem is to cry and withdraw. A key word in the vignette is "suddenly." That this change was abrupt is critical information for developing our hypotheses. A sudden change in her attitude and behavior can lead to speculation that something uncomfortable and possibly traumatic has occurred. Her difficulty in responding to questions about her behavior would add fuel to the notion that something frightening has happened and that she is withdrawing from it. These are some of the hypotheses for the clinician to explore. Others might be the following:

1. The girl is being intimidated by someone at school.
2. An abrupt change has occurred at home and she wants to be there.
3. She is developing a school phobia.
4. She is depressed and her school difficulties are symptomatic of her depression.
5. She has a physical problem that she is afraid to talk about.

These hypotheses provide the therapist with possible explanations for the changes in her behavior. They give direction for further inquiry, but are not intended to be a complete list. Hypotheses help to narrow our focus and rule out possibilities.

Once a few hypotheses have been developed, the therapist can begin to think about what additional information might prove helpful. Being curious about a client can be a useful, nonevaluative position for the therapist's inquiry. Similarly, consultations with supervisors and colleagues can suggest directions to take and questions to pursue. In addition, even preliminary information may suggest the need for referrals for physical examinations, psychological testing, or developmental evaluation.

3

The Initial Interview

It is 5 minutes to the hour when she looks anxiously at the clock, just before the first session. For what feels like the thousandth time, she mentally rehearses exactly what she wants to say at the beginning of the session. She is worried that she will forget something important because of nervousness. She desperately wants to make a good impression. It is now 2 minutes to the hour—if only the butterflies in her stomach would disappear, she might feel ready. She looks at the door, and wishes for a brief second that she could leave. She takes a deep breath as the door to the therapy office opens. . . .

Did you imagine this to be the client or the therapist waiting for the first session to begin? Either could be true. For therapist and clients alike, beginning therapy can elicit feelings of fear, excitement, and nervous anticipation. Each client will take you on a different journey. This chapter will cover the basic issues that must be addressed in the initial interview to ensure that your journey begins with a good start.

DEVELOPING A CONNECTION: HOW TO JOIN WITH CLIENTS

The most crucial task in the first session is for you to successfully join with your clients. *Joining* means that clients feel a sense of connectedness with you, which usually arises when they feel that you understand, respect, and care about them. The importance of joining cannot be overstated: It is the foundation for future work. Failure to successfully join with your clients will hamper all of your efforts, from assessment to treatment. For example, clients will be reluctant to share sensitive information if you have not established a safe and secure relationship with them. Likewise, clients may become highly resistant to or defensive toward suggestions if you have not created a strong therapeutic relationship with them. Ultimately, failure to join with clients will likely lead to premature termination of therapy.

Joining is a process that should be carefully attended to throughout the entire initial interview. It begins in the first moments of therapy, as clients are welcomed into your office. You should attempt to put your clients at ease, since they are most likely anxious about coming to therapy. You might engage in some social talk with them to break the ice before discussing problems. You might ask them what kind of work they do, or what they like to do for fun. Besides making your clients feel comfortable talking with you, this approach demonstrates your personal interest in them. You might also share some information about yourself so that the clients can get to know you. Ideally, you will be able to identify something you have in common with your clients that will help develop a sense of connection.

Joining can also take place at other points throughout the initial interview. For example, joining can occur when you respectfully listen to and address questions your clients have about confidentiality, fees, and other issues. Likewise, giving each of your clients an opportunity to tell his or her story during assessment can facilitate joining by allowing each person to feel heard and understood. Reflective listening, maintaining direct eye contact, or leaning forward can also reinforce to your client that you are interested in and concerned about what he or she is saying. Concluding therapy with a positive message for your clients can be another way to strengthen your connection. For example, a husband who resists coming to therapy can be complimented for caring enough about his relationship to come despite his strong reservations about therapy.

Although skills to facilitate joining can be learned, it is important to recognize that developing a relationship with another person cannot be reduced to a recipe or set of techniques. In fact, the greatest asset any therapist brings to the process is him- or herself. Your personality, attitudes, life experiences, and mannerisms become a part of and help create the relationship.

Although the therapist's personality is usually an asset to promoting joining, there are times when therapist characteristics can create a barrier to developing a connection. Therapists who have prejudices or negative preconceptions about people based on race, ethnicity, sexual orientation, socioeconomic status, or religious orientation will likely have difficulty establishing a connection with clients who have these characteristics. Likewise, therapists may have a difficult time joining with a client who reminds them of someone with whom they had a painful relationship (perhaps a parent or spouse). Therefore, you should be vigilant in assuring that personal issues or prejudices do not interfere with you developing a relationship with your clients.

ESTABLISHING CREDIBILITY

Beginning therapists often fear their clients will ask, "How long have you been doing therapy?" Similarly, questions about one's marital status or parenthood may be dreaded by unmarried or childless therapists because all of these questions reflect a key issue that the beginning therapist must frequently deal with in the initial session—the issue of credibility.

In order for clients to have hope or an expectancy of change, they must see the therapist and therapy as credible, or they may prematurely terminate therapy, if they begin at all. Therefore, it is important for you to assess early on any issues of credibility that need to be addressed. First, do the clients see therapy as an effective way to solve problems? Or do they believe that therapy is only for crazy people? Second, do the clients see you, in your role as therapist, as being competent or credible? Clients may question a therapist's ability to help them because he or she looks too young, or a parent may question a childless therapist's ability to understand and help.

If you suspect there is a credibility problem, you should attempt to pinpoint where and why credibility is lacking. For example, one beginning therapist described how a woman came into the first session saying that she wanted a gay or lesbian counselor. The therapist indicated that she was not a lesbian, and that she had very few friends who were either gay or lesbian. However, she expressed a willingness to learn more about these issues. At the end of the session, when the therapist asked how the woman felt about continuing in therapy with her, given her desire for a gay or lesbian counselor, the woman indicated she was quite comfortable about continuing with the therapist. Through further discussion, the therapist discovered that what initially had appeared to be concern about the therapist's experience working with gay or lesbian issues was actually a fear on the client's part that she would be unfairly judged by a "straight" person. When the therapist expressed an open and accepting stance toward the woman, she was able to earn the client's trust and respect. The more precise your understanding of why the client does not see you or the therapy as credible, the more likely your intervention will be on target in addressing this issue.

In cases where clients are resistant to therapy in general, you may be able to reframe the process in a way that builds its credibility. For individuals who think therapy is only for crazy people, you must work to reduce the stigma. You can compare therapy to coaching, in that even the best athletes, such as Olympians or professionals, use coaches. Therapy also could be compared to consulting work, with clients likened to businesses that hire someone with special expertise to help them.

When clients question a specific therapist's credibility, they usually focus on the lack of some critical professional or life experience. Often you can redefine for the client what type of experience is needed to be helpful. For example, a parent may doubt a therapist's ability to be helpful if he has not parented children of his own. In this instance, the therapist may be able to build credibility by discussing other types of experience working with children (e.g., taking care of a relative's children, or having been a teacher or childcare worker). Alternatively, the therapist may state that in working with several families in therapy, he or she has learned through experience what works and doesn't work in parenting.

In some cases, you can let the client know about your lack of experience in a particular area and then discuss how you can compensate for this limitation. You might indicate that your cases are supervised by a more experienced clinician, or you may ask the client to offer his or her expertise. For example, a therapist can ask clients of a different race or ethnic background to educate him or her about important cultural differences as they arise. Likewise, parents could be told that they are the experts on their children. Thus, the parents' intimate knowledge of their children plus the therapist's experience with families in general will increase the likelihood of therapy being successful.

If clients still harbor doubts, a frequently effective strategy is to contract with them for a set number of sessions (perhaps three). This gives you time to demonstrate your competency. You can explain to your clients that if they are still uncertain about your ability to help them after the agreed-upon number of sessions, you will gladly refer them elsewhere. Nearly all clients are willing to give you this chance, provided the number of sessions is reasonable. In these situations, you need to identify a problem that can be quickly resolved to build credibility with your clients.

It is important that you not become defensive if your credibility is being questioned. If you can deal with your client's concerns in a nondefensive and respectful manner, you may actually build credibility. In order to do this, however, you must be clear in your own mind what you do have to offer, even if you have limited clinical or life experience.

First, you need to recognize that clients value having someone compassionately and respectfully listen to them at a difficult time in their lives. Part of the reason that clients' problems are so distressing to them is that they feel isolated, lonely, and inadequate in relation to others. The therapeutic relationship can provide a sense of connection and support for clients at a time when these essentials are in short supply. For some clients, the relationship with the therapist may be their first healthy relationship, and this aspect alone can be quite therapeutic. In simply being present with another human being, you have something important to offer your clients.

Second, you can frequently offer important insights to your clients because you do not have the kind of emotional involvement in the situation that they do. As an outside observer, you may help illuminate for your clients important aspects of themselves or their relationships with others that can facilitate change.

Third, even the inexperienced therapist has access to clinical knowledge that most clients do not possess or could not easily assess. Through course work preparation, you have learned important concepts and theories that you may use to inform your work, thereby tapping into a source of practical knowledge and wisdom beyond your years of actual clinical experience.

DEFINING CLIENT EXPECTATIONS FOR THERAPY

Another important task in the initial interview is to define client expectations for what therapy will accomplish and how it will proceed, in order to ensure that clients' needs are compatible with what you as therapist can or are willing to offer. In some cases, you may determine that you are not the appropriate therapist for the clients, and you will need to make a referral. In addition, client goals must be integrated with therapist goals to develop an effective treatment plan, which is discussed in Chapter 5.

Defining Client Goals for Therapy

The first step in defining expectations is to ask your clients what they would like to accomplish through therapy. An effective way to introduce this subject is simply to ask questions such as "How can I be helpful to you?" or "What are you hiring me to do?" In many cases, your clients will be able to give you a straightforward answer, such as "Teach us how to better communicate with one another."

In defining goals for therapy, a number of problems can arise. Often, your clients may identify multiple problem areas, with little distinction of priorities. For example, many couples may have a "laundry list" of complaints about each other or their relationship. In these cases, you will need to obtain your clients' perspective on the relative importance of their problems. For example, you might ask, "Of the issues you have presented, which is most and which is least important?"

In other cases, your clients may not have a clear idea of what the problem is or what their goals for therapy are. In these situations you may need to contract for a limited number of sessions to explore and define problem areas and goals. Another potential problem is that clients may have unrealistically high expectations or goals. For example, some individuals may believe that their relationship should be totally free from any conflict. In these cases you may want to validate the client's goal and then reframe it so that it is more realistic and obtainable.

Further, setting goals may be complicated by the unstated agenda of a client, an aim that he or she feels it is not appropriate to disclose. For example, a couple may come into therapy with the stated goal of working on the marriage. Later you may discover that the husband entered therapy to make sure you would take care of his wife after he informed her of his intention to leave the marriage. Sometimes, even the clients may not be totally aware of their reasons for seeking therapy. For example, a divorced woman was eventually able to recognize that she probably was not invested in working on the relationship with her husband when they first entered couple therapy. Rather, she acknowledged that her motivation to try marital counseling was probably a desire to alleviate feelings of guilt about ending the marriage.

Alternatively, spouses and family members may define goals that initially appear incompatible. In these situations, you may need to creatively reframe the goals in such a way as to make them compatible or link them together. For example, parents may want to see their adolescent behave in a more mature and responsible manner, while the adolescent wants greater freedom. A therapist could potentially link these goals together by discussing how both the parents and adolescent have a common desire to see the adolescent become successfully launched as an adult, also pointing out that becoming an adult carries with it certain privileges as well as responsibilities. The therapist can then work with the family to help the adolescent achieve more freedom and privileges consistent with his or her ability to manage responsibility.

Another common scenario involves one partner wanting to make the relationship work, while the other individual seriously contemplates divorce. One possible approach is to suggest the need to evaluate the relationship much like a house inspector would go through a structure to determine which areas have strengths and which areas need attention. To the partner invested in the marriage, the marital evaluation could be explained as a necessary step in determining what needs to changed if the marriage is to be saved. To the partner seriously considering divorce, the marital evaluation can be presented as a means of illuminating why this marriage failed and of helping the individual to avoid making a similar mistake in future relationships if the couple does divorce.

Once you have a clear understanding of what your clients want or expect from therapy, you need to decide whether or not it is appropriate for you to treat the case. First, you must assess whether the case is inside your scope of practice, that is, whether the clients are expecting help for issues that would be considered appropriate for a family therapist to treat. For example, offering legal or medical advice would not be within your scope of practice, but working with a couple on their marriage obviously would be. In many cases, the scope of practice may be defined for therapists by states (e.g., California) that license or certify family therapists. If the case falls outside your scope of practice, you would need to be able to refer your clients to an appropriate professional.

Second, you need to assess the degree to which the case falls within your scope of competence. In other words, do you have the necessary skills, training, or experience to effectively treat the issues? If not, you may need to refer the clients to another therapist who has the appropriate skills or qualifications. For example, a referral would be necessary if your client wanted hypnosis but you did not have any training or experience with the technique. In some cases, you may be able to treat the case provided you take appropriate measures to gain the necessary competence while treating the case. For example, a therapist who has never worked with encopresis could do a literature review on treating this condition and seek supervision on the case.

On rare occasions, the client's goals for therapy may be so incongruent with your own values that you may need to make a referral. For example, most therapists would be uncomfortable helping a client achieve the goal of convincing the partner that having extramarital affairs should be allowed in the relationship. Similarly, a pro-life therapist may have difficulty working with a client who is trying to decide whether or not to have an abortion.

Additional Expectations for Therapy

Many clients not only bring in expectations about *what* therapy will accomplish, but also about *how* therapy will do so. For example, clients who have had previous therapy may assume you will do therapy in a similar manner. If the previous therapist assigned homework, your client may also expect that of you. Whenever a client has had previous therapy, it is generally quite helpful to explore what that experience was like, as it can strongly shape (both positively and negatively) a client's expectations regarding therapy.

You need to explore with your clients what they expect to happen in therapy on a number of dimensions, including how long therapy will be or who will be involved in it. Some clients may expect therapy to be only one or two sessions, while others may expect the process to last a year or more. Likewise, an individual who expects to be seen alone may be surprised when you ask him or her to invite other family members to therapy. Clients can also have expectations about their level of involvement or that of the therapist. For example, some parents bring a troubled child to therapy with the expectation that the therapist will "fix" the child with little involvement on their part. Others expect to be an active part of the therapy process. It is critical to spell out the nature of the therapy at the outset.

You must also assess whether client expectations will impede the therapeutic process. For example, one couple stated that they did not want to look at family of origin issues since they felt this had been unproductive in previous therapy. Yet many of the couple's concerns seemed intimately tied to difficulties with their parents. In a case like this, you would need to determine how rigid the couple is in their desire to avoid family of origin exploration. If they persist in this stance, you would have to decide how flexible you were willing to be to accommodate their desire. In some instances, you may decide against continuing therapy because the expectations are too restrictive and would severely limit your ability to be effective.

BUILDING MOTIVATION

Much of the previous discussion has assumed that clients have some voluntary interest in coming to therapy. Although many clients are motivated, you may quickly discover that not everyone willingly comes to therapy or seeks change. Some clients come to therapy because they have been mandated by the courts to do so because of substance abuse, juvenile delinquency, child abuse, or other issues. Other clients are brought in by their spouses, and adolescents may be compelled by their parents to go to therapy. Although the therapist cannot motivate everyone, there are strategies for assessing and building motivation.

When assessing motivation, it is helpful to conceptualize it as existing on a continuum from high to low. A client's overall level of motivation will be based on a number of factors, assessment of which can guide you in choosing interventions that increase motivation.

A logical time to assess motivation is when defining goals for therapy. Answers to the question "What brings you to therapy?" will differentiate motivated from unmotivated clients. The former usually respond by describing the problems or growth areas they would like to see addressed. If a client responds by saying that someone asked or insisted he or she come to therapy, problems with motivation may be anticipated. For example, a husband may say he came to therapy because his wife threatened to divorce him if he didn't participate. Others may be referred by the courts. Nevertheless, some of these clients can become quite committed to therapy as they experience its benefits in their lives.

You should also inquire who first suggested therapy or called for the appointment. Generally this person is the most motivated for therapy. You might also ask your clients what led them to come to therapy now, rather than sooner or later in their lives? The answer may provide clues to your clients' motivation, as well as important assessment information, such as precipitating events.

Clients will have little motivation for therapy if they do not believe there is a problem, or if they feel that the problem is not serious. You will need to carefully assess whether a problem does indeed exist, and, if it does, why the clients refuse to acknowledge it. You may need to educate a client about the problem and the possible negative consequences of not addressing it. For example, you might warn a client that a failure to heed a partner's complaints could lead to the eventual breakup of the relationship.

Sometimes clients will deny that a problem exists out of fear of consequences, change, or injury to their self-image. Child molesters will frequently deny or minimize the molestation to avoid legal consequences as well as to sidestep admitting to themselves that they are child molesters. In these cases, building motivation for therapy will be entwined with working with the client's denial.

If a mandated client refuses to acknowledge that a problem exists, you can suggest that there is at least one—he or she is being told to come to unwanted therapy. If your client agrees (which is typically the case), then you can explore what needs to happen so that therapy can be successfully terminated. This approach allows you to join with your client, but at the same time work on intermediate goals that address the problem.

Some clients may have poor motivation because they do not anticipate any benefit from therapy, believing that therapy is useless or the situation is hopeless. For some, creating an expectancy of hope will help build motivation. Noting exceptions to the problem might begin to instill some hope. Or a positive experience in therapy during the initial session might spark hope. Of course, feelings of hopelessness and lack of motivation could be a symptom of depression. As this condition is treated through medication or other interventions, depressed clients frequently develop more energy and enthusiasm for therapy.

Other factors might also reduce clients' motivation for therapy. For example, there may be psychological barriers to therapy, such as a client having difficulty trusting others. Some clients may have practical barriers, such as difficulties with transportation, finances, or work schedules.

Using these strategies does not guarantee client motivation. You may still have a poorly motivated client, particularly in court-ordered cases in which the client can avoid prosecution by participating in therapy (for example, cases of sexual abuse or battering). In these situations, you need to become comfortable with using the leverage for change provided by the courts. For example, you may need to inform the client that therapy will be terminated and reported to the courts unless satisfactory progress is maintained.

HANDLING ADMINISTRATIVE ISSUES

One of the remaining tasks in an initial interview is to address issues such as confidentiality and therapy fees. Although these matters are typically called "administrative" issues, it is important to recognize that therapeutic issues are frequently played out through them. For example, one client who was adamant about not being videotaped was discovered through further assessment to have a high level of distrust for people, which became a key area of focus in therapy. Therefore, the therapist who is attuned to the process and not just the content when handling administrative issues may discover important opportunities for assessment or even intervention.

Confidentiality and Release of Information

You should always address the issue of confidentiality with your clients. They need to be informed not only of the confidential nature of therapy, but also of the possible circumstances in which confidentiality will be broken (including duty to warn and child abuse). As discussed in Chapter 2, information on confidentiality may be included on a client information form that can be mailed to clients prior to the first session, or read by them in the office before the first session.

Therapeutic issues may arise when discussing confidentiality with clients. For example, if a husband or wife in couple therapy inquires if the court can obtain therapy records, you might suspect that one of the partners is seriously thinking of divorce.

You will frequently want to consult with other individuals or institutions connected with particular cases, such as previous therapists, psychiatrists or physicians, school officials or teachers, lawyers, courts, and parole officers. In these cases, you will need to have clients sign a release of information form, such as the one depicted in Figure 3.1, to permit communication between you and the other parties. The signatures of all participants in therapy are required for the release of information. For example, you should obtain both the husband's and wife's signatures if both have been participants in the course of therapy.

Videotaping and Observation

Beginning family therapists are frequently instructed to videotape all or some of their sessions for supervision purposes. The vast majority of clients agree to be videotaped if they are approached properly about it. Explain why the videotaping is beneficial to both therapist and client, and address issues of confidentiality regarding videotaping. You can tell your clients that you regularly consult with other therapists, and that videotaping allows them to witness firsthand what happened in therapy. You can then explain that consulting with therapists in this manner is helpful to both you and your clients since "two heads are better than one." You

---

To: _____
(practitioner, hospital, etc.)

I have been informed that under _____ (state) law, communications between a patient and his or her therapist are privileged and may not be disclosed by the therapist unless the patient consents. I also have been informed that patient records maintained by a therapist may not be disclosed to third parties except with the patient's consent or through legal process.

Please check one of the following:

____ I hereby authorize you to provide copies of all my patient records to _____ _____ (primary care physician, other health care professional, insurance company). I further authorize you to discuss my case, including my history, treatment, and condition, with _____ (primary care physician, other health care professional, insurance company).

____ This authorization is only for the limited purpose of releasing information to and discussing my case with _____ (specify). It shall not be deemed a waiver of any privileged communications or confidential information to anyone other than _____ (specify).

This authorization shall remain in effect until revoked by me in writing.

This _____ day of _____, 19 _____.

_____
Signature

_____ _____/_____/_____
Witnessed by   Date

FIGURE 3.1. Authorization for release of information of records.

can add that videotaping allows you to review what happened in previous sessions and perhaps have a new insight, much like people notice something new when watching a movie for the second time. Finally, point out that videotaping the session allows the couple or family to see how they interact when they watch a replay.

You should inform the client of who will view the videotape emphasizing that the videotapes are considered confidential information. Indicate as well what will happen to the tapes after the completion of therapy, assuring clients that videotapes are not permanently kept, but are regularly erased or recorded over. Clients should be asked to sign a form giving their consent for videotaping. The form should outline the purpose of the videotaping, who will view the videotape, and what will happen to the tapes after therapy is completed.

In a small number of cases, clients may be reluctant to be videotaped. You should carefully explore with them their reasons. In many cases, clients may simply be hesitant due to self-consciousness. Most of these clients will be agreeable to being videotaped if assured that theirs is a common reaction and that people generally forget about the camera in a short time. You should pay careful attention to clients who are insistent about not being videotaped since they are the exception rather than the rule. These clients often have sensitive information that they wish to protect or keep secret. For example, one client who refused to be videotaped disclosed indirectly that he had engaged in illegal activities. In some cases, clients will agree to be videotaped if you will turn off the video camera when they indicate that they are ready to disclose particularly sensitive information. If a client is not open to videotaping under any circumstances, you should respect this decision in order to avoid damaging the therapeutic relationship and possible precipitating a premature termination of therapy. Clients may agree to be videotaped once they have established greater trust in you or the therapeutic process.

If therapy will include live supervision or the use of observing/reflecting teams, discuss this with your clients. Most of them will agree to this format if they are told why the supervision or team benefits both therapist and client. It is often helpful to allow clients, at their request, to meet supervisors or team members who observe the sessions from behind the one-way mirror.

Fees

In addition to setting the fee, you should discuss acceptable forms of payment, when the fee should be paid, and fee for late cancellation or "no-show" appointments, if applicable. Figure 3.2 illustrates one version of a payment agreement that contains some of this essential information.

If a third party is responsible for payment, their terms for payment should be clearly understood by therapist and client. Often third party payers limit the number of sessions, or the type of presenting problem or diagnoses they will reimburse. For example, almost no third party payer will reimburse for marriage counseling. Many third party payers will not pay for therapy to treat personality disorders or "problems of living" such as those listed in the "V" codes of the fourth edition of the *Diagnostic and Statistical Manual of Mental Disorders* (DSM-IV; American Psychiatric Association, 1994). If a third party payer is involved, the therapist should verify insurance coverage at the outset of therapy. Issues concerning provider eligibility, annual deductible, rate of reimbursement, and limitations on the number of sessions and types of treatments covered need to be addressed. Usually a DSM-IV diagnosis will need to be assigned to the insured patient.

As with other administrative issues, working out the details for payment can be diagnostic and help to clarify the family's expectations of and responsibilities for therapy. In discussing fees you might learn, for example, that a client is unable to pay the full therapy fee due to specific hardships, such as medical expenses. Alternatively, a client's unwillingness to pay the full therapy fee may reflect low motivation for therapy, a strong sense

---

Professional fees are based on $_____ for a standard _____-minute session. Psychological assessments, consultations, and reports are billed at $_____ per hour. Brief professional services are billed at $_____ per 15 minutes, or any part thereof, including telephone conversations. Fees may be periodically adjusted and clients will be notified in advance of the adjustment.

Professional fees will be assessed at the rate of $_____ per hour, or any part thereof, for any services related to litigation, defense, or other court- or case-related activities. Such activities include interviews, evaluations, research, reports, correspondence, testimony, communication with attorneys, travel, and on-site time. In case of overnight travel, the maximum daily rate will be $_____. Incidental expenses for professional services, such as, but not limited to, cost of travel, lodging, and meals, will be billed to the client or his or her attorney.

Payment in full is expected at the time or in advance of services rendered. Statements will be provided for filing insurance claims. Nonpayment of fees will result in termination of professional services and collection activity for amounts owed.

Since professional services are available only through prior scheduling, sessions canceled less than 24 hours in advance are charged at the full rate of the scheduled service.

Any variation from this payment agreement will require a separate written agreement.

I have read this agreement and agree to its terms.

_____	_____	__/__/__
Client	Guarantor (if different)	Date

_____	__/__/__
Witness	Date

FIGURE 3.2. Payment agreement.

of entitlement, or a victim mentality. Generally, free services tend not to be valued by clients. A fee provides some incentive to make effective use of services.

It is difficult to assign a monetary value to therapy, and therapists often feel uneasy about charging fees while acting in a helping role. Therapist anxiety about fees can easily be transferred to clients and can create conflict and stress in therapy. Comfort in handling fees will increase with therapeutic experience and confidence in your ability to provide a worthwhile service.

Other Administrative Issues

Several other administrative issues need to be addressed with clients. In some cases, therapists may be required to discuss with clients their professional qualifications. For example, California requires by law that all unlicensed family therapists identify themselves to their clients as trainees or interns. Many agencies and practitioners have clients read and sign an informed consent statement that summarizes many of the issues discussed in this chapter. The statement may address issues of confidentiality and payment of fees, and generally includes a brief description of what therapy is, including the potential risks, such as being asked to examine painful issues. Permission to videotape may be included in this or a separate statement. Figure 3.3 is a basic informed consent form that covers some of these issues.

CONCLUSION: THE FIRST SESSION AND BEYOND

The initial interview is a critical time in the therapy process, several important tasks must be accomplished to ensure that therapy will proceed successfully. Developing a connection and establishing credibility with your clients is essential for their return for a second session. Defining expectations for therapy and building motivation are also crucial, as well as properly handling administrative issues.

Clearly, many of the issues discussed in this chapter are important throughout therapy, not just in the first interview. You need to remain connected or joined with your clients in order to effectively confront and challenge them at all stages. Likewise, the goals or expectations for therapy may need to be redefined as therapy proceeds.

I understand that treatment at _____
(Name of treatment facility here)

may involve discussing relationship, psychological, and/or emotional issues that may at times be distressing. However, I also understand that this process is intended to help me personally and with relationships. I am aware of alternative treatment facilities available to me.

My therapist has answered all of my questions about treatment at the _____
(Name of treatment facility here)

satisfactorily. If I have further questions, I understand that my therapist will either answer them or find answers for me. I understand that I may leave therapy at any time, although I have been informed that this is best accomplished in consultation with the therapist.

I understand that at _____:
(Name of treatment facility here)

(a) doctoral students in family therapy conduct therapy under the close supervision of the family therapy faculty.

(b) therapy sessions are routinely videotaped and/or observed by other _____
therapists and supervisors, and
(Name of treatment facility here)

(c) research is part of the ongoing nature of _____.
(Name of treatment facility here)

I agree to allow information from my testing to be included in the ongoing pool of research data, understanding that this material will not contain my name or other identifying information. I further agree to have my sessions videotaped for therapeutic supervision purposes. I understand that videotapes are erased at the end of my treatment unless I have signed the lower part of this form.

To be signed by all participating members.

Signed:_____ Date:_____

_____ _____

_____ _____

_____ _____

_____ _____

_____ _____

I further give permission for videotapes of my therapy sessions to be used for educational and/or research purposes, with the understanding that such tapes will be considered confidential, will have identifying names edited out, and that these tapes will be shown to family therapy professionals and students only.

Signed:_____ Date:_____

_____ _____

_____ _____

_____ _____

_____ _____

_____ _____

FIGURE 3.3. Basic informed consent form.

4

Guidelines for
Conducting Assessment

This chapter presents a plan for approaching assessment. Beginning therapists may easily feel overwhelmed by the amount of information that needs to be gathered in the first few interviews. In an attempt to clarify the assessment process and make it less daunting, we have broken it down into various components and presented them in a logical sequence. However, the reality is that the various areas overlap, and that assessment seldom proceeds in such a straightforward manner.

Table 4.1 shows the general outline for conducting a comprehensive assessment. The initial assessment typically begins by exploring with clients their problems or concerns, and the solutions that have been attempted. At this early stage, you must also assess if your clients are in crisis, or if any possible issues of harm are relevant. For example, a client who is depressed or hopeless must be assessed for suicide. You must also be alert to possible signs of abuse or violence toward others. Since alcohol and substance abuse are commonly associated with relationship problems, they can impede effective treatment if overlooked. In addition, problems may have an underlying biological component which must be ruled out. This chapter also covers the various areas that are important to consider within a general psychosocial assessment, including assessing the individual, the couple or family system, the social systems outside the family, and larger social systems such as culture and gender socialization.

This chapter provides guidelines for conducting a comprehensive assessment within each of these areas. Such a thorough assessment will help you arrive at a more accurate picture of your client and thereby develop an effective treatment plan.

TABLE 4.1. General Assessment Plan

1. Conduct initial assessment.
   - Explore presenting problems.
   - Assess for attempted solutions.
   - Assess for crisis and stressful life events.

2. Rule out potential issues of harm.
   - Assess for suicide.
   - Assess for family violence and abuse.
   - Assess for sexual abuse.
   - Assess for duty-to-warn issues.

3. Rule out possible substance abuse.

4. Rule out possible biological problems.

5. Conduct general psychosocial assessment.
   - Assess affect, behavior, and cognitions.
   - Assess meaning system.
   - Assess spirituality.
   - Assess the couple and family system.
   - Assess social systems outside the family.
   - Assess families within the larger social context.

INITIAL ASSESSMENT

Exploring the Presenting Problems

The problems that bring clients to therapy, the presenting problems, are explored first. For example, you will want to know the nature or description of the problem—what it is, and how long it has existed. You might also inquire about who is most affected by the problem. Is it only manifested at a certain time or in a certain place? You also need to know whom the family conceptualizes as having the problem. Is the problem seen as being a relational one ("We don't know how to communicate"), or is it seen as primarily one individual's problem ("Our child is having difficulty")? When only one person is identified as having the problem, this person is often referred to as the "identified patient" or "IP."

When a single IP is identified, you need to listen for and explore problems other family members may have. This has a twofold purpose. First, it helps you develop some possible hypotheses regarding family dynamics. For example, a family may initially present with a child who has problems at home or at school. With further exploration, you may discover the couple's relationship is conflictual, leading to a possible hypothesis that the child is acting out because he or she is triangulated in the couple's conflict. Second, the family is more likely to understand the justification for family therapy in lieu of individual therapy with the IP if you can successfully highlight other problems within the family system. Obviously, the more invested the family is in having an IP, the more cautiously you will need to proceed.

You should also find out who else knows about or is involved in the problem. This information can help you assess what areas of functioning have been affected by it. For example, you may learn that a child is having difficulties at school if the family discloses that a teacher knows about the problem, or you may discover that your clients are involved in the legal system. In all of these cases, you would be wise to consider getting a release of information from your clients so you can talk with others who may be knowledgeable about the problem. This can also help you assess what resources or social support the clients have. For example, a couple may mention talking to their minister or parents for advice on marital difficulties. In some cases, you may want to include some of these individuals in the treatment plan. You may solicit a teacher's help when dealing with a child's school-related problems, or parents of adult children might be invited in to deal with important family of origin issues.

Finally, it is often enlightening to ask the clients why they think the problem exists. Their insights in this area can help you develop hypotheses. It is not uncommon for one spouse to have good insights on what issues the other partner might need to look at, and vice versa. What is usually missing is insight regarding one's own issues or contributions to the problem. Likewise, ask the clients what others have said about why the problem exists. Again, this information can provide a valuable starting point for you to build hypotheses.

Some therapists from a solution-focused approach believe that a detailed knowledge of the problem is not always necessary to discover solutions or exceptions to the problem. Although this may indeed be true in many cases, therapists need to recognize that having clients tell us their stories (even if problem-saturated) can have value in other ways. For example, respectfully listening can help the client develop a connection with the therapist. In their eagerness to get to solutions and exceptions, we have seen some beginning therapists prematurely cut off clients. Therapists need to be careful about pushing too quickly for solutions, or they risk appearing disrespectful of clients' need to tell their story.

Assessing for Attempted Solutions

In addition to exploring the problems, it is frequently helpful to assess what solutions your clients have either attempted or considered. You thereby can avoid recommending solutions that have been unsuccessfully tried by your clients, which could damage your credibility. You should also explore what solutions your clients have considered but not tried, as well as solutions others have suggested. You can then explore with the clients why they didn't try particular solutions. This often provides you with good information about potential barriers to or negative consequences of change. Another reason to explore attempted solutions is that in some cases they may contribute to or exacerbate the problem (Fisch, Weakland, & Segal, 1985). For example, a husband who withdraws to avoid conflict may actually create conflict with his partner because she interprets his withdrawal as a lack of caring. The therapist may recognize a pattern in a client's attempt to solve the problem and suggest that he or she take a completely different approach.

When assessing attempted solutions, it is extremely helpful to explore if therapy has been tried before. If so, you can explore what was helpful and not helpful about that experience, enabling you to build on past successes or avoid making similar mistakes. You may want to consider recommending books or giving homework assignments if your clients indicate that these were particularly helpful in the past. It would also be wise to explore why the clients are no longer seeing the previous therapist. Did the clients or therapist move, necessitating a change? Or do your clients have a history of working with therapists a short time and then dropping out of treatment? This information will help you assess the likelihood that therapy will have a positive outcome.

Assessing for Crisis and Stressful Life Events

During the initial assessment you should assess the extent to which your clients may be in crisis. Is there a specific event bringing them into therapy, or has there been a pile-up of life events that has created stress? These life events could be of a personal nature (e.g., divorce, illness, death of family member) or involve external social, economic, or political events (e.g., layoffs due to recession, immigration forced by economic or social/political hardship). Are the stressors of an acute or chronic nature? To what extent are the life stressors an underlying cause of the presenting problems? What resources do your clients have for coping? Is the stress creating a demand on the clients that exceeds their coping resources? Whenever clients are in crisis, you should also consider assessing for suicide or other potential issues of harm. Chapter 6 discusses how to deal with clients in crisis.

POTENTIAL ISSUES OF HARM

A critical rule of assessment is the need to be constantly vigilant to any possible issues of harm. Issues of potential harm include harm to self (suicide) or others (domestic violence or homicide, child abuse, or sexual abuse). Each of these issues is discussed herein, along with duty-to-warn considerations.

Suicide

Research on suicide suggests that the majority of people who kill themselves have told someone about their plan in the months preceding the suicide. This person may be a family member or friend, or may be a physician or therapist. Family therapists work with depressed clients on a daily basis and always must be alert for signs that a client is considering suicide.

Many new therapists bring to their first clinical experiences misperceptions about suicide. Two common ones are the notion that discussing thoughts of suicide may cause an attempt on the client's part, and discounting the seriousness of suicide threats, especially when others perceive them as an attempt to get attention or some other goal. Other common misperceptions include the beliefs that a therapist cannot intervene effectively with a client who has decided to commit suicide or that people who commit suicide really want to die.

People who kill themselves frequently are ambivalent about dying. It is usually after a series of unrelenting losses and failures, with little or no relief or hope, that a client finally chooses suicide. Even after making the decision, many suicidal people leave open a way to be rescued. For example, the writer Sylvia Plath, after several failed suicide attempts, was aware that rescue was possible from her final attempt. She turned on the gas in her stove to kill herself but knew that her maid would arrive shortly. Unfortunately, on the day of that attempt, the maid was late to work and Sylvia Plath died.

Assessing for suicide is a therapeutic skill that all beginning therapists should learn. Research has suggested there are certain demographic factors and warning signals that should alert the therapist to the possibility of client suicide attempts. Table 4.2 reflects the demographics of suicide, while Table 4.3 provides a list of danger signs that indicate suicide risk.

In assessing for suicide, the therapist may begin by simply asking the client if he or she is thinking about killing himself or herself. In listening to the client's reply the therapist should assess (1) detail or specificity in the plan (is there mention of a method, time and date, or a planned or written suicide note?); (2) lethality and reversibility (e.g., shooting vs. cutting oneself); (3) intentionality (providing for the possibility of rescue); and (4) proximity (whether important support people know of the plan, are nearby, and express care or concern for the client). The therapist should also assess the same factors in any previous suicide attempts. Additional

TABLE 4.2. Demographics of Suicide

Features	Trends and comments
Age	Suicide rises with age. The increase is linear in white males and peaks at about 50 in females. There has been a recent increase in adolescent and youth suicide.
Sex	More males commit suicide. More females attempt suicide. Recent statistics show rises in suicide rates among young white females.
Ethnicity	More whites commit suicide than nonwhites. Recent statistics show an increase in young black males ages 15–35.
Childhood loss	Early loss is associated with completed suicide, later loss with attempted suicide. Early loss is also associated with scientific and artistic creativity.
Recent loss	The more irrevocable the loss, the greater the risk of suicide. Suicide is associated with an accumulation of losses throughout life.
Alcoholism	Alcohol is associated with high risk of suicide. Treatment for drinking and suicide problems have many features in common.
Mental illness	Suicide is mostly associated with depressive illness.
Physical illness	Suicide is associated with declining health and potency.
Downward economic mobility	Unemployment, frequent job changes, and a trend toward lower status and lower-paying jobs are traditionally associated with male risk, but are no longer sex-linked characteristics.
Living in the center city	Areas of high crime, alcoholism, mental illness, poverty, and family disorganization are associated with social isolation and alienation.
Marital disruption, including divorce, widowhood, and the breaking up of a love affair	The more final the change, the more serious the risk. Marriage is more a protection against suicide for males. Women can survive the loss of a husband better than men can survive the loss of a wife.
Previous suicide attempts	People who have attempted suicide are in a high-risk group. The more serious the previous attempts, the greater the rate of subsequent completed suicide.
History of attempted or completed suicide in relatives and other important figures.	Family members' suicide is associated with a higher risk, as suicide tends to run in families.
A "death trend"	An accumulation of losses and death are a risk factor, and therefore a major reason for relieving the severe death anxiety in the family.

Note. Data from Hirschfeld and Russell (1997).

TABLE 4.3. Warning Signs of Suicide

Features	Manifestations and comments
1. Quiet, withdrawn, few friends	Often not recognized because the individual is not noticed and makes no obvious trouble. Associated with social and family isolation.
2. Changes in behavior	Personality changes, for example, from friendliness to withdrawal and lack of communication, sad and expressionless appearance; from a quiet demeanor to acting out and trouble making. The important thing is the change.
3. Increased failure or role strain	Often pervasive in school, work, home, friends, and love relationships, but often manifested most clearly in school pressures.
4. a. Recent family changes	a. Illness, job loss, increased drinking by the parents or other family members. Often the background of the crisis.
b. Recent loss of a family member	b. Death, divorce, separation, or someone leaving home.
5. Feelings of despair and hopelessness	Shows itself in many forms, from changes in posture and behavior to verbal expression of such feelings. Hopelessness is even more closely associated with suicide than depression.
6. Symptomatic acts	Taking unnecessary risks, becoming involved in drinking and drug abuse, becoming inappropriately aggressive or submissive. Giving away possessions. Associated with changes in behavior.
7. Communication of suicidal thoughts or feelings	Such statements as "Life is not worth living," "I'm finished," "Done for," "I might as well be dead," or "I wish I was dead." Best understood in the context of life changes and family changes.
8. Presence of a plan	Storing up medication, buying a gun. The meaning of these acts and communication can best be understood by sensitive responding to and questioning of the suicidal person.
9. Negative or fearful attitudes toward treatment or psychiatrists	"Shows you're crazy," "It's the end of the road," "I'll end up in the crazy house," and so on. Refusal of help. Associated with conflicts over family loyalties.
10. Impasse in therapy	"Sabotaging" of the therapy, extreme resistance, becoming increasingly depressed or suicidal. Known as the "negative therapeutic reaction," it is often associated with success in therapy and threats to the status quo. Also part of a potentially positive therapeutic crisis.

Note. Data from Hirschfeld and Russell (1997).

risk factors include psychiatric diagnosis, antisocial or borderline personality disorders, substance use, sense of urgency, poor impulse control, poor reality testing, serious medical illness, and life stress.

In addition, the assessment should examine or discover what would prevent the person from committing suicide. In essence, the therapist wants to know what would give the person hope. For example, a divorced, unemployed woman stated that the only reason she did not commit suicide was the pain it would cause her children. The therapist realized that the client was in so much pain that no amount of talk about caring for herself would change her mind. However, her sense of duty and love for her children combined with her religious beliefs about suicide served as strong enough deterrents to keep her alive until her living situation improved. Therapists can listen to and reinforce reasons their clients have for not killing themselves.

Discussing the suicidal ideation or suicide attempts of an individual in front of other family members involves important considerations. The therapist should determine what role family members may serve in preventing or increasing the possibility of a member attempting suicide. For example, sometimes family members threaten suicide when they perceive the possibility of rejection or abandonment by another family member (as in divorce). Intense family conflict can be the precipitating event in an adolescent's suicide attempt. On the other hand, the desire to protect young children from harm can be the only reason a parent stays alive. One client family lost a 16-year-old son in a ski accident, causing the mother to go into a deep depression. Two years later the mother reported that the only factor that kept her from a suicide attempt was the desire to protect her 12-year-old daughter from further loss.

The possibility of suicide is often an unstated family secret of which members are aware in varying degrees. Depending on the age, maturity, and relationships of family members, an open discussion of suicide can lift a burden off the family. Social isolation, family history of suicide attempts, and loss of family members through death or separation are predictors of suicide that specifically involve family relations. Relationships among family members are an important consideration in any discussion of suicide.

Assessing for Violence and Abuse

Estimates of family violence suggest that some type of violence occurs in approximately 15–20% of families. Battering is the single major cause of injury to women (Walker, 1979). Violence can take many forms and be inflicted in many different relationships. While spousal abuse and physical abuse of children are probably the most common forms of violence that therapists see, violence against the elderly is becoming increasingly common.

While many warning signs may suggest that some type of violence is occurring within the client family, therapists should also pay attention to their internal responses to the clients. Frequently, students report having a nagging concern about a family member's safety, even when the session is over. Another frequent internal clue is the therapist's sense of fearfulness, intimidation, and concern for personal safety, particularly because many beginning therapists are young and female.

A list of characteristics of battering men and battered women is presented in Table 4.4 (Walker, 1979; Walker & Hooper, 1982). Power and control are primary issues in battering relationships, along with rejection and fear of being abandoned. Emotional dependence and lack of economic options are two reasons wives and children stay in abusive environments. This situation has led to treatment ideas that focus on finding shelter, economic options, and new connections to supportive people and resources for victims.

Although society and the legal system historically have been slower to intervene in violence between two adults, they have been more attentive to cases that involve potential child abuse. This heightened responsiveness to child abuse is most likely in response to the fact that children are less powerful and able to protect themselves than women. Frequently, spousal abuse and child abuse occur in the same families and are perpetrated by a man who was abused himself as a child. Additional predictors of abuse are families who suffer economic hardships and who are isolated from outside support systems. Table 4.5 depicts the differences between abusive and nonabusive families (Thorman, 1980).

When violence is an issue, the therapist can no longer conduct "therapy as usual." Insight into the violence will not protect the victims. Safety of the victims at home and during the therapy sessions is of paramount importance. This means that the therapist must become very practical in his or her treatment approach finding out if the victims can escape and if they have a safe place to go. If the victims are children or elderly and thus unable to protect themselves, the therapist must be even more active, becoming a representative of society by stating unequivocally that the violence must stop immediately and then notifying the proper authorities to ensure that it does.

The switch from client's advocate exploring therapeutic issues to social worker assessing and addressing practical concerns of living and safety to representative of society using one's authority to stop client's behavior can be a difficult process for beginning therapists. Most therapists choose their profession because they want to help people in a col-

TABLE 4.4. Characteristics of Batterers and Battered Women

Characteristics of men who batter	Characteristics of battered women
Low self-esteem.	Low self-esteem.
Believes myths about battering relationships.	Believes myths about battering relationships.
Believes in male supremacy and stereotyped masculine sex role; a traditionalist about the home.	Believes in family unity and prescribed stereotype of the female sex role; a traditionalist.
Blames others for his actions.	Willing to accept responsibility for the batterer's actions.
Is pathologically jealous.	Suffers from guilt while denying the anger and fear she feels.
Presents a dual personality.	Presents a passive personality but has strength to prevent further violence and to prevent being killed.
Has severe stress reactions, which he may use drinking and wife battering to escape.	Has severe stress with psychophysical complaints.
Often uses sex as an act of aggression to enhance self-esteem; may be bisexual.	Uses sex to establish intimacy.
Does not believe his violent behavior should have negative consequences.	Believes no one can help her escape her predicament.
Low frustration tolerance, poor impulse control, explosive temper; external locus of control.	"Martyrlike" behavior.
Emotionally dependent on wife and children.	Emotionally and/or economically dependent on husband.
Family history of domestic violence.	Family history of domestic violence.
Accepts violence as viable method of problem solving and maintaining family intact.	Accepts violence in hopes that she will be able to help husband change; believes she provokes anger and violence.
As a control mechanism, often abuses or threatens children and pets.	Gives in to husband's demands in order to protect children and pets.
Was physically and/or sexually abused as a child or saw "significant other" abused by spouse (usually mother by father).	Was physically and/or sexually abused as child or saw violence at home.
High degree of job dissatisfaction; under- or unemployment, which leads to feelings of inadequacy.	Often employed but not allowed to control finances.
Maintains close contact with his family.	Loses contact with her family due to own embarrassment or forced isolation; may maintain contact with husband's mother.
Unrealistic expectations of relationship.	Traditional expectations of husband as provider and of self as mother and wife.
Preoccupation with weapons.	
Power and control a primary issue.	

TABLE 4.5. Differences between Abusive and Nonabusive Families

	Characteristics of nonabusive families	Characteristics of abusive families
Parenting	Nurturing of child; normal expectations.	Control of child; role reversal with child; child expected to nurture parents; excessive expectations.
Family relations	Clear boundaries; autonomy encouraged.	Blurred, confused boundaries; autonomy discouraged; symbiotic ties of dependency.
Communication	Open and spontaneous verbal expression of feelings, attitudes, and ideas.	Constricted verbal communication; feelings communicated by behavior.
Norms and rules	Flexible rules; internalized controls.	Rigid, inflexible rules; controls enforced from outside (punishment).
Conflict resolution	Conflicts negotiated; communication used to resolve conflicts.	Coercion, force, and violence used to resolve conflicts.

laborative manner. Violence and abuse are two of the infrequent therapeutic situations in which therapists must take an authoritarian stance and insist that a behavior stop.

Assessing for Sexual Abuse

As with violence, sexual abuse occurs more frequently than reported. Although research varies, national surveys indicate that approximately one in five women and one in nine men report being victims of sexual abuse as children (Finkelhor, Hotaling, Lewis, & Smith, 1990). The definition of sexual abuse varies from state to state, but usually it is said to occur when an adult or older child initiates an interaction with a child for the purpose of sexually stimulating or gratifying the perpetrator or other person (Lauer, Lourie, Salus, & Broadhurst, 1979).

Researchers indicate that factors such as duration and severity of sexual abuse influence the effects on the victim (Kilpatrick, 1987). However, all victims do not carry the abuse similarly. Some adults who were victimized in childhood show signs of posttraumatic stress disorder, including recurrent thoughts and emotions and avoiding situations that

remind them of the trauma. Women seeking counseling for sexual dysfunction problems in marriage often report childhood sexual abuse
(McGuire & Wagner, 1978).

The majority of sexual abuse cases involve male perpetrators and
female victims. Abusers commonly live in the same household with the
victim. Biological fathers are more likely to sexually abuse an offspring
than are biological mothers; stepfathers are more likely to abuse stepdaugh-
ters than biological fathers; and a mother's boyfriend or live-in compan-
ion is more prone to abuse the mother's daughter than either a biological
father or stepfather (Gordon & Creighton, 1988).

Perpetrators and victims of childhood sexual maltreatment usually
do not voluntarily self-report; detection is often left to the therapist, who
may be given indirect behaviors as clues. Due to the legal implications of
both physical and sexual abuse, it is vital to handle each case with care,
since specific court testimony might be needed. Limiting the number of
times a child discloses his or her experience is vital for the emotional
welfare of the child.

Using a biopsychosocial perspective, sexual abuse assessment stems
from information about a child's physical condition, behavior, and social
context. If a child indicates several of the following symptoms, further
interviewing needs to be done: (1) physically, a child may display sleep
disturbances, encopresis, or enuresis, complain of abdominal pain, or suffer
from appetite disturbances with corresponding weight change; (2) behaviorally, a child may manifest a sudden, unexplained change in behavior
(anxiety or depression), regressive behavior, or overly sexualized behavior or information given the child's age, or experience suicidal thoughts,
run away, or abuse substances; socially, family conditions include a child's
parentified role, inadequate parental coping skills, marital difficulties leading to one parent seeking physical affection from the child, isolated social
context, alcohol and drug use, and a history of parental sexual abuse
(Edwards & Gil, 1986).

Interviewing possible child abuse victims is an art requiring specialized training and skill development. If child abuse is suspected, the family
therapist will continue to interview if trained to do so, or will refer the
child to a specialist, usually through child protective agencies available in
the community.

Duty-to-Warn Issues

Legal issues are another important concern when either violence or sexual
abuse is suspected or known. In most states, reporting of child neglect,
physical abuse, or sexual abuse is mandated by law. It is imperative that
you know the laws of your state in this regard. Beyond legal knowledge,

one's best clinical judgment will be required in some situations. For example, in most states mandated reporters (which usually include therapists) are required to report suspected abuse. They also are expected to report neglect, which involves the absence of care, in contrast to a specific act, like abuse, that is done to a child.

What constitutes enough evidence to report is a judgment call that most beginning therapists are still developing. When new therapists initially suspect abuse, they should immediately involve their supervisors. Recently, several lawsuits have been initiated by family members who have been accused of abuse that they assert they did not commit. This is especially problematic when the victim is older and the accusations are based on repressed memories that have surfaced in therapy. Therapists are given significant power by the law surrounding abuse issues. The suspicions they have about abuse in a particular family can change the family's life irrevocably. Therapists must be aware of this power and use it as judiciously as possible. This means the therapist (1) is informed about state laws, (2) goes over any suspected abuse case with the supervisor in as timely a manner as possible, and (3) gathers as much information as possible and reports this as clearly as possible.

Gathering information is another skill that therapists develop over time. Particularly when abuse is suspected, the therapist must be careful in eliciting and documenting information. Ideally, the interview could be on videotape, carried out with a supervisor or more experienced therapist, or even just with the "expert" on abuse at the student's placement. The therapist wants to know the who, what, how, where, and why of each situation without asking leading questions or giving responses that might influence what the victim says. The therapist also needs to assess for imminent risk.

States often require that suspected child or elder abuse be reported to the proper authorities, an exception to the legal principles of confidentiality and patient privilege which guide most therapeutic exchanges. Therapists are not legally bound to tell client families that any form of child or elder abuse will be reported, but many therapists choose to make this information known from the beginning of therapy. One way to uniformly tell clients your policies on reporting abuse is to create a handout that they can read in the waiting room before the initial session.

ASSESSING FOR SUBSTANCE ABUSE

Substance abuse is one of the major mental health problems in the United States. In fact, many health care payer groups single out substance abuse as a separate budget item. Although some experts assert that there is a substance abuse epidemic, abuse and addictions are commonly overlooked in therapy unless the substance problem is the presenting problem.

Therapists overlook abuse issues for a variety of reasons. First, the clients may not consider the abuse to be a problem itself, but, rather, the result of some other issue: a bad job, painful childhood, or conflictual marriage. Clients come to therapy asking for help with the "problem" and fail to mention their substance abuse. The therapist might collude by failing to ask about use of substances, or drug and alcohol abuse might be overlooked because there is no clear definition of when a social drinker becomes a problem drinker or when the latter becomes an alcoholic. In other words, the abuser might not view his or her substance use as problematic. The family may consider the substance use a problem but be afraid to mention it.

One of the authors had a client family report that the father could not be an alcoholic because he only drank beer. Families have different definitions about what constitutes a substance abuse problem. Is dependence on caffeine an addiction? Is recreational use of marijuana a problem? When does regular substance use become a problem? Experts do not agree on these issues, and neither do families. Even if families believe that a member's substance abuse is a problem, they often collude to hide it from the therapist.

For example, a therapist had as clients a couple who defined the wife's presenting problem as the husband's drinking. The husband's presenting problem was the wife's nagging, particularly about his drinking. The therapist presented the following three different theories to the couple and suggested that the goal of therapy was to decide which theory was true (1) Alcohol abuse by the husband is the problem; (2) conflict about the alcohol is the problem in the relationship; and (3) the wife's distortions about the alcohol are the problem. He then challenged the husband to quit drinking for 2 weeks to help discern "the truth." When the husband could not quit drinking, he became willing to consider the first theory.

The most common mistake new therapists make regarding substance abuse is to overlook the possibility of it. Substance abuse is frequently comordid with, that is, it exists along with, other disorders such as depression or anxiety. It also is associated with violence, abuse, automobile accidents, homicides, and suicide. It is essential to know the variety of ways substance-abusing clients can present in therapy. The second step is to routinely ask about substance use in initial interviews with new clients.

There are several commonly used screening tests for assessing alcohol abuse (Kitchens, 1994). Questions raised in these tests could be asked about substances other than alcohol. Two frequently used tests are the Michigan Alcoholism Screening Test (MAST) and the Alcohol Use Disorders Identification Test (AUDIT), depicted in Figures 4.1 and 4.2, respectively. The MAST has been widely used and has been examined with generally favorable results in terms of reliability and accuracy. It is made up of 24 yes/no questions and scoring indicates the subject's degree of alcohol dependence. Shorter versions of the MAST have also been developed. The AUDIT questionnaire is much shorter but has less data on reliability and validity.

Points	Questions
2	1. Do you feel you are a normal drinker?
2	2. Have you ever awakened the morning after some drinking the night before and found that you could not remember a part of the evening before?
1	3. Does your spouse or parents ever worry or complain about your drinking?
2	4. Can you stop drinking without a struggle after one or two drinks?
1	5. Do you ever feel bad about your drinking?
2	6. Do friends or relatives think you are a normal drinker?
2	7. Are you always able to stop drinking when you want to?
5	8. Have you ever attended a meeting of Alcoholics Anonymous?
1	9. Have you gotten into fights when drinking?
2	10. Has drinking ever created problems with you and your spouse?
2	11. Has your spouse or other family member ever gone to anyone for help about your drinking?
2	12. Have you ever lost friends or girlfriends/boyfriends because of your drinking?
2	13. Have you ever gotten into trouble at work because of drinking?
2	14. Have you ever lost a job because of drinking?
2	15. Have you ever neglected your obligations, your family, or your work for two or more days in a row because you were drinking?
1	16. Do you ever drink before noon?
2	17. Have you ever been told you have liver trouble? Cirrhosis?
2	18. Have you ever had delirium tremens (DTs), severe shaking, heard voices, or seen things that weren't there after heavy drinking?
5	19. Have you ever gone to anyone for help about your drinking?
5	20. Have you ever been in a hospital because of your drinking?
2	21. Have you ever been a patient in a psychiatric hospital or on a psychiatric ward of a general hospital where drinking was part of the problem?
2	22. Have you ever been seen at a psychiatric or mental health clinic or gone to a doctor, social worker, or clergyman for help with an emotional problem in which drinking had played a part?
2	23. Have you ever been arrested, even for a few hours, because of drunk behavior?
2	24. Have you ever been arrested for drunk driving or driving after drinking?

FIGURE 4.1. Michigan Alcoholism Screening Test (MAST). From Selzer (1971). Copyright 1971 by American Psychiatric Association. Reprinted by permission.

The CAGE (Cutting down, Annoying, Guilt, Eye-opener) question-naire (Ewing, 1984) consists of four questions: "(1) Have you ever felt you ought to cut down on your drinking? (2) Have people annoyed you by criticizing your drinking? (3) Have you ever felt bad or guilty about your drinking? (4) Have you ever had a drink first thing in the morning to steady your nerves or get rid of a hangover (an 'eye opener')?" These

---

1. How often do you have a drink containing alcohol?

| Never | Monthly or less | 2 to 4 times a month | 2 or 3 times a week | 4 or more times a week |

2. How many drinks containing alcohol do you have on a typical day when you are drinking?

| 1 or 2 | 3 or 4 | 5 or 6 | 7 to 9 | 10 or more |

3. How often do you have 6 or more drinks on one occasion?

| Never | Less than monthly | Monthly | Weekly | Daily or almost daily |

4. How often during the last year have you found that you were not able to stop drinking once you had started?

| Never | Less than monthly | Monthly | Weekly | Daily or almost daily |

5. How often during the last year have you failed to do what was expected from you because of drinking?

| Never | Less than monthly | Monthly | Weekly | Daily or almost daily |

6. How often during the last year have you needed a first drink in the morning to get yourself going after a heavy drinking session?

| Never | Less than monthly | Monthly | Weekly | Daily or almost daily |

7. How often in the last year have you had a feeling of guilt or remorse after drinking?

| Never | Less than monthly | Monthly | Weekly | Daily or almost daily |

8. How often during the last year have you been unable to remember what happened the night before because you had been drinking?

| Never | Less than monthly | Monthly | Weekly | Daily or almost daily |

9. Have you or someone else been injured as a result of your drinking?

| No | Yes, but not in the last year | Yes, during the last year |

10. Has a relative or friend or a doctor or other health worker been concerned about your drinking or suggested you cut down?

| No | Yes, but not in the last year | Yes, during the last year |

FIGURE 4.2. Alcohol Use Disorders Identification Test (AUDIT). From Saunders, Aasland, Babor, De La Fuente, and Grant (1993). Copyright 1993 by The Society for the Study of Addiction to Alcohol and Other Drugs, Carfax Publishing Ltd., Abingdon, UK. Reprinted by permission.

simple questions can be memorized and integrated with a regular intake interview.

The CAGE questionnaire has been tested for accuracy in several different settings. Generally, a positive response to two or more questions identifies a problem drinker. Frequency is another key variable in the assessment of a substance problem. Other behaviors that might indicate a substance problem include the amount of substance used in one setting, the reasons the client uses the substance, and what happens when the client tries to stop using the substance.

ASSESSING FOR BIOLOGICAL FACTORS

George Gershwin spent several years in psychoanalysis with an analyst who had two medical degrees. When he finally died, an autopsy found a brain tumor that explained his aberrant behavior. To avoid making the same mistake as Gershwin's analyst, family therapists must consider biological or organic factors in assessment. Unfortunately, the reality is that family therapists are trained to recognize and treat psychological and social problems and frequently have limited knowledge of biological influences. Thus, we run the risk of misinterpreting important clues to a possible biological problem as a symptom of something we have been trained to treat— interpersonal problems. However, being mindful of this risk can help prevent overlooking possible biological or organic factors.

An awareness of biological problems does not require that you be an expert in human physiology. However, therapists must recognize the telltale signs of an underlying biological problem and also recognize that psychological symptoms do not necessarily imply psychological causes (Taylor, 1990). You also need sensitivity to any information that seems outside the usual content of a family therapy session. Instead of dismissing the unusual content because it does not fit with one's model, a therapist needs an attitude of openness and curiosity to pursue a line of questioning wherever it may lead, including to a referral.

Therapists should be aware of several clues that might indicate biological problems, including (1) no history of similar symptoms; (2) no readily identifiable cause; (3) age 55 or older; (4) chronic physical disease; and (5) drug use. Other clues suggest the possibility of organic brain disease. Symptoms of a brain syndrome might result from a brain tumor, seizures, heart disease, or liver failure. One or more of the following cognitive deficits suggest a brain syndrome: inattention, disorientation, recent memory impairment, diminished reasoning, and sensory indiscrimination. Other clues suggesting a brain syndrome include head injury, changes in headache pattern, visual disturbances, speech deficits, abnormal body movements, and alterations in consciousness. The more clues there are, the more suspicious you should be. These clues should alert you to begin a different line of questioning, focusing on the individual and his or her symptoms. Other family members may be asked to corroborate details given by the IP or to give their own impressions. Discovery of these symptoms should lead you to make a prompt referral for medical evaluation. Document this referral in the client's record and note the reasons the referral was made.

An important diagnostic tool that family therapists should be familiar with is the Mental Status Exam (MSE). MSEs are used frequently by physicians during physical exams as a rapid assessment tool to detect changes in orientation, intellectual functioning (language, memory, and calculation), thought content, judgment, mood, and behavior. MSEs are used less frequently in family therapy, perhaps because most clients who come for family treatment do not demonstrate any behaviors that would raise concerns about intellectual functioning.

While it is probably prudent to refer a client to a physician if unusual symptoms (such as those listed earlier) are noted, you can conduct an MSE immediately and obtain information that will be helpful in making a referral. When doing a MSE, the therapist should consider the client's appearance, the interaction, the client's awareness of where he or she is and what he or she is doing, appropriateness of behavior, the client's mood, use of language, attention and concentration, short- and long-term memory, ability to perform simple calculations and answer specific questions, the presence of delusions (bizarre thoughts) with or without hallucinations, social and moral judgment, and impulsiveness (Dilsaver, 1990). Figure 4.3 provides a sample of some of the factors considered during a thorough MSE, while Figure 4.4 includes a number of questions that can be asked in a brief mental status check.

A short mnemonic to remember the elements of a mental status exam is JOIMAT: judgment, orientation, intellectual functioning, memory, affect, thought processing. A family therapist may perform MSEs so infrequently that it is difficult to remember the details of the exam. However, by memorizing the mnemonic and asking oneself "What is unusual about this client and what questions should I ask to obtain more information?" you can begin investigating possible biological etiologies to problems. For example, an elderly couple was receiving supportive family therapy in conjunction with the husband's treatment for lung cancer, which was in remission. During one session the husband seemed confused and unable to focus. The therapist wondered if these behaviors were cognitive symptoms of depression, a normal response to cancer. However, the therapist referred the husband back to his physician, and a CT scan was done, with the results indicating that the cancer had spread to his brain.

GENERAL PSYCHOSOCIAL ASSESSMENT

Psychopathology and the ABCs:
Assessing Affect, Behavior, and Cognition

Most psychological theories focus on affect, behaviors, or cognitions. As a result, both assessment and treatment goals usually address one of these domains. We believe that all good clinicians attend to affect, behavior,

1. Is the client's appearance unusual?
2. Is the nature and quality of the client's interaction with the examining therapist and others (such as family members or friends) appropriate?
3. Is the client oriented to person, place, and time? (orientation to time includes the ability to specify the month, the day of the month, the day of the week, the year, and the season of the year)?
4. Is the client oriented to the circumstances? Does the client understand the nature of the therapist/client relationship and have an appropriate manner?
5. What is the client's affect (predominant emotional tone)?
6. What is the client's mood (reported emotional state)? Is the reported mood congruent with therapist's perception of affect?
7. Is there evidence of an abnormality in the sphere of language? Consider rate, intonation, modulation, nonverbal gestures and expressions, and whether these are congruent with content. Is there evidence of aphasia?
8. Is the content of the client's thought noteworthy? Is there evidence of delusions, obsessions, or unnecessary worry or phobias?
9. Is there abnormality in any of the five senses? Are there reports of hallucinations or delusions?
10. Are the client's attention and concentration impaired?
11. Are defects in short- or long-term memory reported or detected on formal examination of these abilities?
12. Is the client's social and moral judgment within the limits of his or her cultural group?
13. Does the client have suicidal or homicidal ideation or intent? Does the client have the means to carry out any plans to harm self or others? What is the client's level of impulse control?
14. Can the client perform calculations with the speed and accuracy expected of someone with the same educational and occupational background?
15. Is the client properly oriented in space? Does the client distinguish between right and left?
16. Does the client have the sense of direction that is expected? (Are there reports of getting lost when traveling repeated routes?)
17. Is the client's ability to think abstractly commensurate with his or her educational background?
18. Can the client copy geometric figures?

FIGURE 4.3. Some factors considered during a mental status exam. Adapted from Dilsaver (1990). Copyright 1990 by American Academy of Family Physicians. Adapted by permission.

and cognitions regardless of their theoretical orientation. A key reason to assess in all three domains is that symptom descriptions for mental disorders in DSM-IV usually fall into one of these categories.

Certain disorders of childhood, such as oppositional defiant disorder and conduct disorder, focus almost exclusively on behaviors, while delusional disorder focuses on patients' beliefs about themselves or their relationships, and mood disorders primarily involve changes in emotion and affect. Symptom lists for most DSM-IV disorders address all three domains, although the focus varies by disorder. In recent years, DSM editors have tried to remove the theory-driven terminology (e.g., such phrases as "defense mechanisms") and instead use observable criteria. These changes should make it easier to do an assessment of the patient's symptoms.

During your assessment, consider whether the problems the client describes and those you observe fit more into one category than another. You can consider the "ABCs" as well as whether the symptoms cluster together in a way that match a DSM-IV diagnosis, although family systems theory usually describes interaction, not individual symptoms (Denton, Patterson, & Van Meir, 1997). It is not necessary to be a purist, choosing an exclusive focus on family interaction or individual diag-

1. What is the date today?
2. What day of the week is it?
3. What is the name of this place?
4. What is your telephone number (or address)?
5. How old are you?
6. When were you born?
7. Who is the President of the United States now?
8. Who was the President just before that?
9. What was your mother's maiden name?
10. Subtract 3 from 20 and keep subtracting 3 from each new number you get, all the way down.

For clients with high school education:

    0–2 errors = intact mental function

    3–4 errors = mild mental impairment

    5–7 errors = moderate mental impairment

    8–10 errors = severe mental impairment

Allow one more error if the client has only a grade school education. Allow one less error if the client has education beyond high school.

FIGURE 4.4. Short Mental Status Questionnaire. Adapted from Dilsaver (1990) and Pfeiffer (1975). Copyright 1990 by American Academy of Family Physicians. Adapted by permission.

nosis—using both frameworks can lead to the most complete assessment picture.

It is important that you have a basic understanding of DSM-IV because it represents the common language shared by mental health clinicians. In addition, many treatment methods and psychopharmacological remedies are tied to DSM-IV individual diagnostic categories. While you may not have memorized criteria for every possible diagnosis, you should be able to recognize depression, anxiety, substance abuse, somatization, and other common disorders. Cultivate an attitude of curiosity, and think of yourself as a keen observer of the human condition. Write down a list of the most salient symptoms your patient describes, and note your own observations along with the nature of your interaction with the client. Then ask yourself, do these symptoms cluster in a way that fits a DSM-IV diagnostic category? Consider also the possibility that your patient may demonstrate more than one disorder; comorbidity is common.

Assessing for Meaning

One of the most important aspects of assessment is to understand the meaning system that each client attaches to the issues presented in therapy. The meaning system is essentially composed of the various cognitions, beliefs, memories, and emotions that a client consciously or unconsciously uses to make sense or out of his or her daily experiences. The meaning system influences how the individual views and interprets internal and external experiences, and how he or she chooses to respond to those experiences.

It will be difficult for you to create change without understanding how your clients make meaning out of their experiences. In one case, a woman with a chronic illness became upset whenever her husband offered any type of advice regarding her illness. She accused him of being very unsupportive of her and her illness, and was threatening to leave the relationship. He in turn was hurt and confused by this accusation because he felt he was expressing concern whenever he suggested things to her. By exploring the meaning that the woman ascribed to her husband's advice giving, the therapist discovered that she interpreted his advice as evidence that he thought her chronic illness could be cured. She feared that once he truly discovered that her illness was chronic and not curable, he would perceive her as a burden and leave. This opened the door to discussing important issues in the relationship regarding illness, caretaking, and trust.

You can use a variety of approaches to understanding or mapping the client's meaning system. Usually the best approach is to ask your client directly what meaning he or she attributes to something. However, this approach is not infallible. In order to trust your client's self-report, you must have confidence that your client is being honest, is cooperative, and is sufficiently self-aware. Clients are not always willing or capable of this. For example, child molesters may be unwilling to fully disclose details or even admit to molesting a child out of shame or fear of legal consequences. In some cases, clients may have little psychological insight to their motives or reasons for doing things. To the extent that we all have some psychological processes that operate outside of our immediate awareness, client self-report has some limitations.

In addition to self-reports, you can sometimes infer aspects of your client's meaning system based on his or her observable behavior and the context in which that behavior happens. When a husband silently withdraws after his wife criticizes him, the inference can be made that the husband was hurt by the remark. The difficulty with making inferences based on behaviors is that several alternate meanings are possible, raising the possibility that an incorrect inference will be made. This risk is evident when working with distressed couples; partners frequently attribute a more negative intent to their partner's behavior than the partner intended.

Your knowledge in specific content areas can also be an important aid in inferring how information is processed by each individual. For example, a good grounding in human development can help you understand an adolescent's behavior in the context of his or her need for independence. Likewise, understanding a client's cultural background may provide important insights into the differences in an individual's interpretations of certain behaviors or events, as compared to the dominant culture.

Assessing Spirituality

One of the most crucial areas that therapists often overlook in their assessment of meaning is the client's religious or spiritual life (Bergin, 1991). Therapists have been reluctant to address spiritual issues for several reasons. For one, many therapists were trained during a time when the scientific–empirical epistemology was held in highest esteem. During their training, therapists learned that if it can't be measured, it shouldn't be considered in assessment. In addition, conducting an assessment implies the possibility of treatment. Most therapists would consider themselves unable to provide spiritual solutions or treatment and would perhaps equate any spiritual treatment as a form of proselytizing.

Bergin (1991) encourages psychotherapists to consider spiritual issues as part of psychotherapy by noting that a spiritual perspective can strongly contribute to a client's (and therapist's) view of human nature, morality, and rituals and practices. In addition, he points out that thera-pists' lack of recognition of religious and spiritual practices is largely at odds with the beliefs of the clients they treat. The general public is more religious, and more often bases life on religious tenets, than psychothera-pists do (Bergin, 1991). For example, a recent Gallup Poll found that 50% of elderly people surveyed said they wanted their doctors to pray with them as they faced death, while 75% said that physicians (and therapists) should address spiritual issues as part of their care (Connell, 1995).

When assessing spiritual issues, you can conceptualize your role as one of asking open-ended questions, assuming a position of curiosity about your client's beliefs, and seeking simply to understand your client's story (Griffith & Griffith, 1994). For example, you can ask yourself, "In what ways and for how long has this patient's life been changed as a result of spiritual beliefs and experiences?" The spiritual experience need not be dramatic for a genuine "conversion" in terms of a changed life to occur.

Several models for spiritual assessment and research instruments have been developed in the last 20 years (Fitchett, 1993). Fitchett's 7 × 7 model for spiritual assessment is one example of such an assessment guide (see Figure 4.5). Many of these models focus on understanding how spiritual beliefs or practices serve a person rather than on examining specifically what the beliefs and practices are. These models view spirituality as a multidimensional process. Regardless of one's assessment approach, spiri-tuality is best seen as a complement to mental health assessment. It "does not displace the accumulated empirical knowledge of mental functioning and mental health treatment" (Bergin, 1991, p. 399).

Assessing the Couple and Family System

One of the things that distinguishes family therapy is the importance it places on assessing the couple or family system in order to place the indi-vidual in proper context. Obviously, the theoretical lens that you use will influence your assessment approach with couples and families. For ex-ample, a Structural family therapist may see enmeshment or diffuse bound-aries, whereas a Bowenian therapist may see fusion or an undifferenti-ated ego mass within the same family. However, they each tap into an underlying concept of closeness or distance. Thus, our approach in this section is to outline important areas of assessment to consider regardless of which theoretical orientation you choose. The specific way in which these issues are explored will depend on your personal style as well as your theoretical orientation. Chapter 5 discusses in more detail how a theo-retical perspective can be integrated into both assessment and developing a treatment plan.

Holistic Assessment

1. **Biological (medical) dimension:** What significant medical problems has the person had in the past? What problems do they have now? What treatment is the person receiving?

2. **Psychological dimension:** Are there any significant psychological problems? Are they being treated? If so, how?

3. **Family systems dimension:** Are there at present, or have there been in the past, patterns within the person's relationships with other family members which have contributed to or perpetuated present problems?

4. **Psychosocial dimension:** What is the history of the person's life, including place of birth and childhood home, family of origin, education, work history, and other important activities and relationships? What is the person's present living situation and what are the person's financial resources?

5. **Ethnic, racial, or cultural dimension:** What is the person's racial, ethnic, or cultural background? How does it contribute to the person's way of addressing any current concerns?

6. **Social issues dimension:** Are the present problems of the person created by or compounded by larger social problems or dysfunctions of which the person is largely a victim? If the person is in part suffering from larger social problems can they become aware of them and join with others in efforts to address those problems?

7. **Spiritual dimension**

Spiritual Assessment

1. **Belief and meaning:** What beliefs does the person have which give meaning and purpose to their life? What major symbols reflect or express meaning for this person? What is the person's story? Are there any current problems which have a specific meaning or alter established meaning? Is the person presently or have they in the past been affiliated with a formal system of belief (i.e., church)?

2. **Vocation and obligations:** Do the person's beliefs and sense of meanings in life create a sense of duty, vocation, calling, or moral obligation? Will any current problems cause conflict or compromise in their perception of their ability to fulfill these duties? Are any current problems viewed as a sacrifice or atonement or otherwise essential to this person's sense of duty?

3. **Experience and emotion:** What direct contacts with the sacred or divine or with the demonic has the person had? What emotions or moods are predominately associated with these contacts and with the person's beliefs, meaning in life, and associated sense of vocation?

4. **Courage and growth:** Must the meaning of new experience, including any current problems, be fit into existing beliefs and symbols? Can the person let go of existing beliefs and symbols in order to allow new ones to emerge?

5. **Ritual and practice:** What are the rituals and practices associated with the person's beliefs and meaning in life? Will current problems, if any, cause a change in the rituals or practices they feel they require or in their ability to perform or participate in those which are important to them?

6. **Community:** Is the person part of one or more formal or informal communities of shared belief, meaning in life, ritual or practice? What is the style of the person's participation in these communities?

7. **Authority and guidance:** Where does the person find the authority for their beliefs, meaning in life, for their vocation, their rituals and practices? When faced with doubt, confusion, tragedy, or conflict, where do they look for guidance? To what extent does the person look outside themselves or inside themselves for guidance?

FIGURE 4.5. Fitchett's 7 × 7 model for spiritual assessment. Adapted from Fitchett (1993). Copyright 1993 by Journal of Pastoral Care Publications. Adapted by permission.

Family Structure

The first step in the family assessment process is to obtain the family structure. If you are interested in multigenerational issues, the family structure assessment ideally should include at least three generations (e.g., child, parent, and grandparents). A genogram (McGoldrick & Gerson, 1985) is a convenient way in which visually capture the family structure. The family structure should reflect all the individuals who are significant in the client's life either by their presence or their absence. For example, the family structure should include both biological parents even if the client has little or no contact with one of them, because the absence of a parent is often a therapeutic issue. Likewise, the family structure should not be restricted to biologically related relatives since other people, such as stepparents and live-in nannies, can have a significant influence on a client's life. Asking about multiple marriages and who lives with whom is often helpful in uncovering significant individuals who may not be biologically related.

The family structure can be an important source of clinical hypotheses. You could explore possible loyalty conflicts that may exist in a remarried family constellation, or discuss how a single parent without proper social support may be overwhelmed with parenting responsibilities. Likewise, hypotheses could also be generated based on the sibling constellation (birth order, gender, age difference of siblings). For example, a first-born child may be more likely to be parentified.

Life Cycle Issues

You should also consider life cycle issues when conducting an assessment. Is the family dealing with particular life transitions, such as birth of the first child or launching children? Is the family having difficulty with these transitions? Conflict between a parent and an adolescent may be related to the adolescent seeking greater autonomy. Or is a child's need for attention being ignored as result of a parent focusing on a new marriage? You should also consider if the life transitions are occurring in the normative range, as well as the possible presence of stressors due to life cycle issues. For example, a couple may be feeling overwhelmed from the demands of caretaking both their own children and elderly parents.

The Couple's Relationship

Assessing the couple's relationship is obviously important when doing marital or couple therapy. However, it is important for you to assess the couple relationship even if the presenting problem centers on a child. Marital or couple conflict can have a significant impact on children. For example, a parent may inappropriately turn to a child to get his or her emotional needs met if the couple relationship is not fulfilling, or a child may act out because he or she is triangulated in the parents' conflict.

A good place to start when doing a couple assessment is to administer a brief marital quality instrument, such as the Marital Adjustment Test (Locke & Wallace, 1959) or the Dyadic Adjustment Scale (Spanier, 1976). These instruments will give you an idea of the overall level of distress in the relationship. In addition, they will quickly help you assess the areas in which the couple is having conflict (e.g., sex, finances, in-laws, etc.) or, conversely, the areas in which the couple is doing well. Among other instruments that provide the clinician with a more detailed assessment of the couple's relationship in a variety of content areas are the Marital Satisfaction Inventory (Synder, 1979) or ENRICH (Fournier, Olson, & Druckman, 1983).

You should also assess for possible issues of commitment. If the couple is not married, is one or both of the individuals ambivalent about continuing the relationship? If the couple is married, has either one seriously considered divorce? Brief pencil-and-paper instruments such as the Marital Instability Index (Edwards, Johnson, & Booth, 1987) or the Marital Status Inventory (Crane, Newfield, & Armstrong, 1984; Weiss & Cerrato, 1980) can be used to measure the likelihood the couple will divorce. You should also assess whether or not one or both individuals may be significantly involved with other people or activities that impact their commitment to a relationship. For example, does one partner, or both, spend a significant amount of time with friends, parents, or children at the expense of time with the partner? Likewise, does the amount of time that one or both partners spend at work or with hobbies negatively impact the relationship?

Assessing how issues of control and responsibility are handled in the relationship is also important. An excellent way to assessing this is to explore how the couple makes decisions. Do they share decisions together, or does one person usually make the decision? Is physical violence or the threat of it used for control (see previous section on issues of harm). Does the couple follow a traditional or an egalitarian model? Have the couple agreed upon their roles and responsibilities within the relationship? Or does one partner overfunction while another partner underfunctions?

The nature of the couple's interactions can also reveal much about their relationship bond. Does the couple do activities together, or do they lead independent lives? What type of activities (e.g., leisure, vacations, projects, attend church, volunteer work, etc.) do they share? To what extent is the couple verbally or physically affectionate with one another? Does the couple have a satisfactory sexual relationship? If not, what are the nature of the concerns? Exploring the couple's courtship can be helpful in assessing relationship bonds. For example, what first attracted the couple to one another? Did the couple have an extremely short or long courtship? In some cases, reviewing the courtship history may uncover that a couple has not properly bonded (e.g., deciding to marry to legitimize an unexpected pregnancy).

You should also assess a couple's communication and conflict resolution skills. In terms of communication, can the couple listen to one another? Can the couple express their thoughts and feelings to one another? In addition, are they able to take responsibility for their own feelings (e.g., using "I" statements), or do they frequently take a blaming stance? Having the couple discuss an issue while you observe their interaction can be an excellent approach to assessing communication skills. In addition, you will want to assess how conflict is handled in the relationship. Is the couple conflict-avoidant? Does the couple ever get physically violent during fights (see issues of harm)? It is also helpful to assess if the fights or conflicts follow a predictable sequence or pattern. Circular questioning (see Chapter 6) can be a particularly effective tool for uncovering the pattern in a couple's fights.

You will also want to explore how children (or the lack of them) impacts the couple's relationship. If the couple does not have children, do they plan to have children? Are there any factors (e.g., infertility, one partner does not want children, etc.) that are keeping them from having children at this time? If the couple has children, are they able to support one another or is parenting a source of conflict for the couple? Even if the couple is no longer married, you should assess the impact of children on the relationship. For example, are the parents engaged in a custody battle, or have they been able to work out an effective coparenting relationship?

Family Assessment

Like couples, families should also be assessed for issues of commitment, control and responsibility, relationship bonds, and communication and conflict resolution skills.

In terms of commitment, you should assess how committed the parent or parents are to their children. In an intact family, are both parents equally invested in parenting? In divorced or separated families, are both parents still involved with the children? If not, why? How has the child or children made sense of this? Do the parents have favorites or certain children with whom they are more invested than others? Is a child being scapegoated for family problems and being forced out of the family? It is also important to explore if one or both parents have other commitments or problems that negatively impact their parenting. For example, are the children's needs being ignored as a parent focuses energy on a new relationship or marriage? Are one or both parents focusing too much energy into work at the expense of their children? Is a mental illness or some other stressor reducing the parent's energy for managing and nurturing children?

You should also assess for possible issues of control and responsibility within the family. Consider how the parents monitor their children's activities and behavior. Assess how discipline is handled. Are the consequences for misbehavior appropriate and administered in a calm or nonreactive manner, or is there evidence of physical abuse (see previous section under issues of harm)? Are the parents consistent in enforcing the rules? You should assess if the children have developmentally appropriate levels of responsibility and privileges. Look at the responsibilities each child has. Is a youngster being parentified? That is, is a child knowledgeable or concerned about issues that would only be appropriate for adults? To what extent are children given age-appropriate input into making decisions?

A third important area to explore is the nature of relationship bonds between family members. Are any parent–child dyads particularly conflictual? Do the parents spend an appropriate amount of time with their children, helping with homework, playing, or other activities? Do the children receive praise from their parents, as well as verbal and physical affection? Do the parents rely too much on their children for their own emotional needs? Is there any evidence of sexual abuse (see issues of harm)?

When exploring the relationship bonds between family members, it is important that you consider other relationships within the family besides those of parent and child. Sibling relationships can be an important source of support for children. In addition, sibling conflict may indicate that the children may be aligned with different parents, who in turn are in conflict with one another. Therefore, you should also assess what type of interactions the children have with one another. Do they do a lot of activities together? Are the relationships generally harmonious or highly conflictual? In multigenerational households, you should also assess the relationships between various family members. For example, does the child have a close or distant relationship with a grandparent who also lives in the household?

Finally, you should observe how family members communicate and resolve conflicts with one another. Are family members able to speak without being interrupted? Do family members speak for one another? Are children comfortable sharing their thoughts, feelings, or fears with their parents? Do family members have difficulty talking about certain topics or issues? Likewise, are certain emotions such as anger or sadness unacceptable to have or to express? Are family members respectful when talking to one another, or are they verbally abusive? Does conflict ever escalate to the point of one or more family members being physically aggressive with each other (see issues of harm)? Do the conflicts seem to follow a repetitive pattern?

Assessing Social Systems Outside the Family

Although as a family therapist you will be primarily concerned with assessing the couple or family system, it is important to recognize that a thorough assessment will also extend beyond these boundaries. Family members interact with a variety of social systems outside the immediate family. For example, the extended family often plays a critical role in the immediate family's life. However, schools, work, friendship networks, and neighborhoods are also important social systems to assess. In other cases, the courts, social service agencies, health and medical services, or other psychotherapists may be involved with one or more family members. A thorough assessment will consider the potential influence that each of these areas may have on the clients.

Assessing these systems outside the immediate family should be carried out with several purposes in mind. First, you should assess if stressors outside the family are contributing to the issues within the family. Stressors from work could be contributing to a couple's difficulties. Likewise, illness or other problems in the extended family could be impacting a family or couple.

Second, you should assess the degree to which individuals or systems outside the family can provide support or resources. Extended family members may be able to provide important emotional or instrumental support. Friends may also be able to provide needed help. If you find that your clients have limited support outside the family, then you may want to work with them to develop a better social support network.

Third, it is important that you assess each family member's level of functioning outside the family. Do family difficulties impact the individual's work performance? Does a child's misbehavior occur primarily at home, or is it present at school as well? Asking questions such as these will help you assess the severity of the problem. In some cases, you may find that a family member has a significantly higher level of functioning in another system—for example, a child may manifest fewer problems at school than at home. In these cases, you can take a solution-focused approach and identify what factors contribute to your client's functioning or well-being in one setting.

Fourth, assessing external systems may provide important clues to individual and interpersonal dynamics within the family. In many cases, individuals may relate to people outside the family in ways similar to how they relate to family members. One client openly discussed his distrust of friends and work colleagues, which in turn illuminated his pattern of interaction with his divorced wife. Carefully assessing family members' interactions with people outside the family can uncover or validate dynamics within the family.

Finally, you should assess the potential impact that systems outside the family can have on the therapy process. Some clients, for example, are mandated to come to therapy by the courts. You will want to be clear on what the courts want to see accomplished, and what the consequences are for noncompliance. In other cases, multiple therapists might be involved with various family members. Ideally, therapists will work closely with one another to avoid working at cross purposes.

Whenever you must work with another individual or system outside the family, the potential always exists for triangles or alliances that may interfere with the therapy process. A couple involved in divorce and a custody battle may each have their own therapist, both of whom need to be careful not to become so strongly aligned with their own client that they simply create a conflictual relationship that mirrors the conflict between the couple. In another case you may need to guard against being triangulated between a school and family over a child's behavior.

Assessing Families within the Larger Social Context

Family therapy has been criticized in the past for ignoring the important influence that historical, social, and economic contexts have on individuals and families (Goldner, 1985; James & McIntyre, 1983; Taggart, 1985). Feminist family therapists have discussed how gender socialization and inequity in society have important implications for how men and women experience family. Just as individually oriented therapists have been said to ignore the family context of a child's misbehavior, family therapists have been accused of ignoring the societal context of family dynamics.

Gender socialization is an important contextual system that should be included in assessment. It is not uncommon for differences in gender socialization to contribute to conflicts between men and women in intimate relationships. In one case, a husband complained that his wife was always checking up on him, which he resented and saw as controlling. The wife insisted that she was simply interested in hearing how his day went, and wasn't checking up on him. She felt distressed over how he angrily withdrew, which resulted in her feeling isolated and alone. This in turn increased her need for connection with her husband. For this couple, gender socialization was contributing to their distance–pursuing cycle. Like many men, the husband was socialized to value independence and be sensitive to issues of status, hierarchy, and control. As a result, he interpreted her "checking in" as "checking up" on him. The couple was able to interrupt the distance–pursuing pattern through a better understanding of how gender socialization was contributing to their cycle.

Like any generalization, however, the therapist needs to recognize that exceptions occur with regard to common gender patterns. Some women may have stereotypical male behaviors or beliefs, while some men may have stereotypical female behaviors or beliefs. Gender patterns should be regarded as hypotheses that need to be confirmed or ruled out with further assessment, not rigidly applied to all male–female dynamics.

When gender socialization is a contributing factor to a problematic dynamic, the therapist will frequently find other factors that reinforce it. For example, the dynamics of an enmeshed family of origin may reinforce the societal message that a woman receives—to take care of others' needs at the expense of her own. In the preceding case example, the husband's fear of control was reinforced by having had a controlling parent. Therefore, you should be aware that factors in addition to gender socialization may reinforce a problematic dynamic.

The racial or ethnic background of a family is also important to consider when doing assessment, particularly if it differs from your own. Sensitivity to culture is critical, beginning with the initial interview. Research shows (Sue & Sue, 1980) that African Americans, Chicanos, Native Americans, and Asian Americans terminate at a significantly higher rate after the first interview than do Anglo clients. Fortunately, respectful and sensitive awareness can instill more confidence in the therapeutic relationship. For example, one of the authors, a 115-pound, middle-class, non-drug-using Caucasian, recalls her first client in her first internship: a 250-pound, tattoo-bearing, heroin-addicted, economically disadvantaged Chicano male nicknamed "Mugs." What developed was a wonderful working relationship, due to the client's willingness to educate the therapist and the therapist's ability to find empathic connections with the client.

Three general guidelines apply to a culturally sensitive assessment. First, you should consider a client's cultural background when interpreting the information gained through assessment. For example, similar behaviors may have different meanings in different cultures (Garbarino & Stott, 1989). In American culture, a child who fails to make eye contact with adults might be perceived to have poor self-esteem. However, in other cultures a child who makes direct eye contact with an adult would be showing disrespect. Likewise, be aware of your own cultural filter, because this will affect how you perceive different clients and their actions. For example, you and your clients may have different expectations regarding appropriate family communication or the way to raise children due to your different cultural backgrounds.

Second, you should not assume that group norms for specific cultural groups will automatically apply to an individual from that group. Therefore, any assumptions about an individual's behavior based on cultural norms must be regarded as tentative until they can be confirmed through further assessment. For example, children from a recently immigrated family may be more acculturated to the American culture than their parents or grandparents. To some degree, each family must be taken as a "case study," since the degree to which a family accepts or displays a cultural prescription is unique to that family.

Third, you should be sensitive to potential power differences between cultural groups. For example, members of a minority group might be reluctant to discuss sensitive information because they fear prejudice from the majority group (Garbarino & Stott, 1989). This in turn can affect a therapist's approach to assessment. Expectations for how therapy can help also need to be explored. Many cultures expect therapists to take on an authoritative role, while others expect more mutuality.

The preceding guidelines for sensitive, cross-cultural assessment can also be applied when exploring cultures that are defined by a characteristic other than race or ethnicity. The *American Heritage Dictionary* (1985) defines culture as "the totality of socially transmitted behavior patterns, arts, beliefs, institutions, and all other products of human work and thought characteristic of a community or population" (p. 348). Note that race or ethnicity is not specifically mentioned. This suggests that we can more broadly conceptualize culture to include social groups or populations based on characteristics such as religious affiliation or sexual orientation. Likewise, cultural differences can be anticipated between individuals who belong to different age cohorts, occupations, social classes, and so forth. Each of these social groups has the potential to influence an individual's sense of identity, beliefs, and manner of relating to others. Therefore, you should determine which of these potential cultures is most salient to each family member and assess for its impact on the family.

However broadly one chooses to define "culture," we need to be reminded that when a family's cultural heritage is positively accessed, a clinician acquires one further resource for change. As Minuchin and Fishman (1981) point out, "Every family has elements in their own culture which, if understood and utilized, can become levers to actualize and expand the family members' behavioral repertoire" (p. 262).

CONCLUSION

In many ways, conducting a thorough assessment is a little like putting a puzzle together. The initial assessment involves putting the corner and edge pieces together first in order to get oriented to the case. Then, you begin to put the rest of the puzzle together piece by piece until a clinical picture emerges. Important pieces of the clinical puzzle include assessing for potential issues of harm, possible substance abuse concerns, and possible biological factors. You must connect these concerns to other pieces of the puzzle, such as possible psychopathology, the clients' meaning system, and issues of spirituality. These pieces in turn must interlock with social systems including couple and family relationships, relationships outside the family, and larger social systems, such as culture and gender socialization. If you address each of these interconnected pieces of the puzzle, we believe that you will obtain a complete clinical picture of your clients.

5

Developing a Treatment Focus

This chapter lays out ways to develop a treatment focus using clinical reasoning. It will help you to organize the assessment information you have obtained over the first few meetings with your clients and to develop a therapeutic contract. The therapeutic contract defines the problems to be addressed in the therapy and the particular interventions that will be offered to address the problems. Writing an initial treatment plan begins to formalize your treatment contract.

After a beginning family therapist learns to "breathe" (that is, make it through the first few sessions of therapy) and begins to join and assess what is going on in the family, the question "Now what do I do?" is heard by supervisors. Clinical reasoning is the process in which you begin to conceptualize, or make sense out of, the problems presented using family therapy theory. It is a time to write down what you do know from the assessment information and to hypothesize about what you do not know. Clinical reasoning provides direction regarding who needs to attend the therapy session, which interventions to use, how long the therapy will last, and whether or not consultation with outside professionals, such as physicians and teachers, will be necessary. All family therapists need to know how to conceptualize and articulate what they do. Developing the capacity to "reason clinically" is essential to becoming proficient in one's professional discipline. This chapter will help you to develop this capacity.

DEVELOPING AN INITIAL TREATMENT PLAN

A treatment plan outlines your focus in the therapy. Therapists are increasingly required to document their work, especially if they are being paid through their clients' insurance carrier. Developing such a plan involves a set of logical steps, as seen in Table 5.1. The first three steps can usually be written after the first one to three meetings with a client. The discipline of writing down an assessment and treatment outline at this juncture can organize treatment significantly.

Step 1 in writing an initial treatment plan involves listing problems that the client presents and the therapist uncovers during the assessment. Especially in the first session, clients express their concerns regarding specific problems they are coming to therapy to manage differently. However, when the therapist conducts a biopsychosocial assessment, other problem areas may be added. For example, a couple might state that they are having difficulty communicating and often escalate into shouting matches. As the therapist assesses when this occurs, he or she may hypothesize that alcohol is a possible contributor to their interaction. Exploring the role of alcohol in the couple's marriage (as well as any multigenerational alcohol patterns) might be added to the problem list.

Step 2 of an initial treatment plan is to include some acknowledgment of the history of the problems presented to you. Previous treatment and experiences in therapy can be useful for the therapist to review. Understanding the current problems as acute or chronic is also part of this process. Clients present or past therapeutic resources can also be noted. Contacting previous therapists (if written permission is given by your client) may provide important information.

Step 3 offers a place for the conceptualization of the case using family therapy frameworks and a diagnostic determination using the DSM-IV multiaxial assessment. Four theoretical family therapy frameworks will be discussed, which systematically interpret a family's presenting problem attempting to explain the causes. Each theoretical framework offers options to help relieve suffering due to the client's depression. Also each framework makes clinical sense, and, after the first few sessions will provide a better fit with problem genesis and resolution than other forms of therapy.

TABLE 5.1. Developing an Initial Treatment Plan

Step 1: Select a problem list.

Step 2: Examine history of problems and previous/current treatment.

Step 3: Conceptualize the case and make a diagnosis using a DSM-IV multiaxial assessment.

Step 4: Establish long-term treatment goals.

Step 5: Select treatment modality, objectives, and interventions.

Step 6: Determine length and frequency of treatment.

Step 7: Consider referrals to outside resources.

Diagnostic determinations according to the DSM-IV multiaxial assessment are another important component in the development of an ongoing treatment plan. These diagnostic determinations are significant since they are used by medical insurance companies in determining reimbursement for therapy sessions.

In Steps 4 and 5, the therapist must determine how he or she will address the problems from the standpoint of family therapy goals and interventions. Basic to writing realistic treatment goals and determining what interventions to use is the family therapist's ability to conceptualize the problem from multiple vantage points. His or her theoretical training becomes essential here. What do we offer to a family that is stuck in troubling interactions? What do we have to offer a suicidal adolescent, or a couple seeking assistance after an affair, or a child who does not want to go to school? Which family members need to be involved in the treatment? Which modality of treatment will we use—will individual, dyadic, family, or group therapy be more effective? Most beginning and many seasoned therapists can become confused here. The section "Conceptualize the Case and Make a Diagnosis Using a DSM-IV Multiaxial Assessment" offers a way to choose clinical problems that family therapists can treat, to use family theory practically to understand one's case, to select interventions that make sense, and to invite significant family members or other persons into the treatment.

Step 6 estimates length of therapy and how often we will be working with the client. Determining if the case is appropriate for crisis, brief, or longer-term treatment needs to be evaluated. Frequency of meetings must also be decided.

Step 7 reminds the family therapist that other professional or community involvement may enhance quality care. Medication referrals or psychological testing can maximize the care we provide.

Outlining the seven steps in an initial treatment plan will focus and clarify your treatment. Try to write one within the first three sessions with your client. If you get stuck, talk through the case with a supervisor or colleague. Several of the following sections detail components of the initial treatment plan, and sample plans follow at the end of the chapter.

SELECT A PROBLEM LIST

The therapist must be able to summarize the presenting problem(s) and to reflect these essential concerns back to the family. For example, if the presenting problem as described by a mother is "too many angry outbursts and running away" by her 14-year-old son, and as described by the son is "getting her off my back," a negotiated definition of the problem by the client system might be "not knowing how to get along when you have differences." If the presenting complaint of one remarried partner is "he spends too much time at work" and of the other is "she is too lenient with her children and too harsh with my children," the negotiated definition of the problem might be "the difficulty blending the styles of two families into one family."

To summarize several family problems, the therapist and the family must negotiate which problem will be handled first, second, and so on. For example, if a family is struggling with agreeing on a parenting style with their adolescent daughter as well as determining if an elderly parent should move in with them, there needs to be a discussion on which of these concerns will be the priority for treatment.

Writing down the agreed upon "problem priority list" begins a formalized treatment plan and helps the therapist and the family stay focused. If the family wants to change the focus of treatment, the therapist can review the list and talk with the family about it. This step is helpful for beginning therapists since one common problem is the "complaint-of-the-week client" who shifts chaotically from topic to topic. Referring to a co-created written list will focus treatment. It can also help the family determine when therapy can be terminated.

Within the first three sessions, you will need to verbally state the negotiated problem list back to the family. If there are several issues, agreement regarding the urgency of each must be made.

EXAMINE HISTORY OF PROBLEMS AND PREVIOUS/CURRENT TREATMENT

An historical perspective regarding problem treatment must be summarized. For instance, a therapist must ascertain if the problem is new or chronic. This can be accomplished by inquiring about a client's previous treatment and experiences in therapy. If a therapist obtains written consent, important information maybe gained by contacting previous therapists. Once the presenting problem is placed within its historical context, a diagnostic determination can be made.

CONCEPTUALIZE THE CASE AND MAKE A DIAGNOSIS USING A DSM-IV MULTIAXIAL ASSESSMENT

In teaching, we have found that beginning family therapists become confused by the "smorgasbord" of available theoretical interpretations used to understand presenting problems. Sometimes schools remedy this by

TABLE 5.2. **Family Therapy Frameworks**

	Historical	Structural	Process	Experiential
Hypothesis on presented problem	Recycled issues from past relationships	Flaws in family structure (hierarchy and boundaries)	Stuck interactional sequences	Unexpressed affect
Specific theories	Transgenerational, object relations, grief therapy	Structural	Strategic/Mental Research Institute, solution-focused, cognitive-behavioral, Milan-systemic, psychoeducational	Experiential, symbolic–expressive, narrative
Founders of theory	Bowen	Minuchin	Haley	Satir, Whitaker
Assessment tools	Genogram, transference and counter-transference	Enactment, family map	Circular questions, hypothesizing	Sculpting, storytelling, restorying
Interventions	Coaching differentiation, detriangling, interpretation, "holding environment", letter writing	Joining, blocking, restructuring, unbalancing, boundary marking	Directives, paradox, exceptions, change reinforcements, contracting, educating, skills training, restorying	Sculpting, self-disclosure, validation, humor, metaphor, psychodrama

teaching only a few theories, causing trainees to miss out on the wonderful variety of family therapy traditions available. The summary in Table 5.2 provides a picture of four broad, theoretical frameworks that can clarify ways to conceptualize cases while still remaining faithful to myriad family therapy theories.

These four theoretical frameworks systemically interpret a family's presenting problem, attempting to explain the cause. Specific family therapy theories associated with each general framework are noted, along with the "founders" of the theories. Finally, although the lists are not at all exhaustive, some assessment and intervention tools are noted under each category.

First, a simple case example will illustrate the process a therapist can use to understand the client's problem conceptually, and then a more in-depth example will be offered. The purpose of this process is to select appropriate goals and interventions that make sense for the therapist and client.

You have met for two sessions with a 19-year-old Caucasian woman who is attending college. She reports the following difficulties: anxiety but no sleep disturbance; ambivalence in her relationship with the young man she has been dating for 3 months; recurrent episodes over the past year of eating large amounts of food in a short period of time, followed by use of laxatives; a fear of becoming "overweight like my Mom, who calls me often to check how I'm doing"; very high expectations of her school performance; friendship with a woman who compulsively exercises and sometimes vomits to control her weight. She has never sought help from professionals before.

You can begin to outline the first three steps of an initial treatment plan. The client presents with several initial problems: anxiety, bulimic eating patterns, and relationship ambivalence. She has never come to therapy before, although she reports that she reads self-help books. From a diagnostic perspective, she would meet criteria for bulimia, while her anxiety symptoms call for further assessment.

The next step is to examine how you might make sense of and treat this young woman from a systemic perspective. Think about the information you have from the case so far. Refer to each of the four family therapy frameworks in Table 5.2 and hypothesize about the presenting problem. Do her symptoms seem to (1) stem from a transgenerational pattern of compulsive behaviors, (2) involve parents who are enmeshed with their daughter, (3) occur after she has had a fight with significant others in her life, or (4) link to feelings of anger or fear that she cannot express?

The four frameworks offer a different systemic understanding of presenting problems or symptoms. The historical framework looks to the past to understand the present. Bowenian and other transgenerational theories as well as object relations therapies fit this framework. One understands the present problems by looking for clues from the past and from the family of origin. In this case, the therapist might first look for a legacy of obesity by developing a genogram with the client.

The three other frameworks look at present interactions for clues about why the presenting problem exists. In the structural framework, we would understand current problems to result from faulty family structure (e.g., boundaries that are enmeshed or disengaged), or from inappropriate hierarchical relationships (e.g., a parentified child). In our case example, the 19-year-old may have been a surrogate spouse for her mother and the enmeshed relationship was threatened when the daughter moved away to school.

The process framework encompasses the majority of theories associated with family therapy—strategic, solution-focused, psychoeducational, communications, as well as cognitive-behavioral and behavioral. Problems stem from interactional patterns that are repeated and are unproductive. Yelling at a child for running away might lead to the child running away more often, which leads to more yelling. In our case example, the client's bingeing behavior might occur after her mother calls or after she has had a negative interaction with her boyfriend, which then leads to further negative interactions, which lead to further binge eating.

Finally, the experiential framework holds that a lack of emotional expression—a person is limited in affective range—often leads to presenting family problems. In our case example, the young woman can show expressions of fear or anxiety, but is limited in her ability to recognize and to express feelings of anger directly within her relationships.

Pause and reflect on one or two of your clinical cases. You can conceptualize each family's presenting problems by using information that you have gained in the first few sessions and by matching it to a theoretical understanding of why these problems are present. This useful exercise will develop your clinical reasoning and will help answer the question "What should I do next?"

To illustrate clinical reasoning more fully and from multiple vantage points, we can consider the following case illustration:

A lower-income, Irish-Catholic 42-year-old woman, married for 22 years with two children, ages 21 and 17, comes into therapy complaining of fatigue, lack of motivation, tearfulness, hopelessness regarding the future of her marriage, a close yet conflictual relationship with her mother, and distress over being laid off from her work as an administrative assistant. The client reports that her husband sometimes drinks too much and has been working part-time and irregularly in construction. They have significantly increased their arguments about money and doing housework. She says her children don't need her like they used to. The 21-year-old son is finishing college and lives out of the home, while the daughter is beginning her senior year of high school. When asked to prioritize the issues, she says that "feeling down and hopeless" is the most pressing matter for her. Although she has felt down at various points in her life, recently she has not wanted to get out of bed, has been unable to sleep, feels worthless, and notes that her family has been expressing worry about her. She had a few counseling sessions several years ago during one of her depressive episodes, but says that she didn't "click" with the therapist. She had briefly talked with her physician, but had not followed through on the doctor's suggestion that medication might help.

Multiple problems can be seen in this case, but the client and therapist agree that working on depressive symptoms is an appropriate place to begin treatment. The therapist can diagnose the major problem as recurrent clinical depression (DSM-IV 296.22). Besides considering possible biological contributors and interventions, the therapist can understand and treat the depression from a family therapy or systemic perspective. Each general family therapy framework can help the therapist conceptualize the client's presenting problem, direct who would be invited into the therapy, and help the therapist choose further assessments and interventions that make sense clinically.

Vantage Point 1: Historical Framework

A historical perspective understands the presenting problem as a recycled issue from the past. Depression stems from unresolved family of origin issues, specifically, the client's lack of differentiation from her own mother. Depression runs in women in the family. The client's recent job loss triggered more severe symptoms of depression; her mother lost a job as she underwent a hysterectomy after the birth of her second child (she had wanted four children) and had suffered from depression then. The mother again suffered from depression at age 42 when her oldest child got married and moved several states away.

- Who should attend therapy?: Client and/or any family members
- Assessment tool: Three-generation genogram (see Figure 5.1)

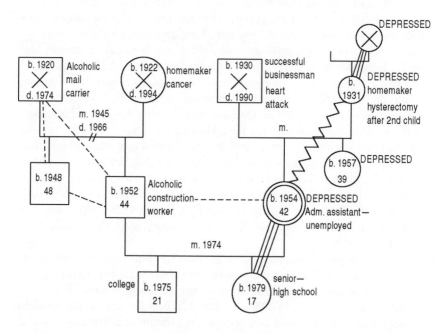

FIGURE 5.1. Case genogram.

- Possible "next step" interventions: Developing and interpreting genogram; writing letter to mother; coaching woman on differentiation by asking her what she would "keep" and "let go of" from her family of origin patterns, especially gender patterns.

Vantage Point 2: Structural Framework

A structural perspective understands the presenting problem as stemming from inappropriate family structure, usually flawed family hierarchy or boundaries. Depression comes from an inappropriate hierarchy, in which the wife is the only parent in the family. The husband's alcoholism and inconsistent work pattern significantly limits his authority. The wife takes care of most household tasks and the parenting of the children, and until recently was the most consistent source of income production. The job loss made this flawed family structure more apparent. Adding to these problems, the client's mother is critical of her when they interact.

- Who should attend therapy?: Client and husband; entire family
- Assessment tools: Joining; enactment of arguments regarding housework and money; enactment of criticism between client and her mother; structural family map (see Figure 5.2).
- Possible "next step" interventions: Restructuring boundaries to have teenager and father take on more household responsibilities so Mom can rest and job-hunt; solidifying diffuse boundary between client and mother by limiting phone contact; creating clearer subsystem boundaries between husband and wife by assigning dates.

Vantage Point 3: Process Perspective

Depression comes from stuck interactional sequences between the client and her husband, especially regarding finances and household work. Depression can also be conceptualized as an "internal" stuck dialogue of cognitions and affect.

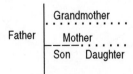

FIGURE 5.2. Structural family map.

- Who should attend therapy?: Client and husband; client individually
- Assessment tools: Circular questioning to understand interaction sequences between the spouses (see Figure 5.3); logged "automatic thoughts" and behaviors in stressful situations (see Figure 5.4)
- Possible "next step" interventions: Exploration of exceptions in sequencing when couple worked together as a team rather than isolating and blaming each other; replacement of automatic "irrational" thoughts with rational thoughts.

Vantage Point 4: Experiential Perspective

Depression develops due to the inability to express anger and fears in the family. Client keeps her feelings to herself and has difficulty identifying and expressing them to family members; husband "drinks" instead of expressing feelings directly.

- Who should attend therapy?: Individuals and/or any combination of all family members
- Assessment tools: Sculpting; family drawings; asking about the family story
- Possible "next step" interventions: Debriefing of sculpting and drawings; identification and expression of feelings directly to others in the family, validation of each person's affect; requesting family members to create the next chapter in their family story.

If the client presents with symptoms meeting the criteria for a mental health diagnosis (usually represented in the DSM-IV), this determination

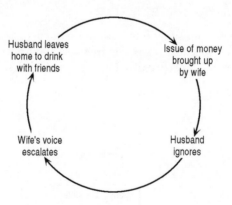

FIGURE 5.3. Interactional sequence.

can be used. "V" codes, such as partner relational problems or parent–child relational problems may be included also. Historically, family therapists have been reserved in adopting a medical model for diagnostic labels in their systemic work. But recent changes in patient care emphasize a biopsychosocial context of understanding human suffering. Medical expertise (the biological component) and social expertise (the relational and contextual component) often combine to relieve psychological symptoms such as depression and anxiety. Family therapy has gained therapeutic recognition in certain domains of medical treatment. In the future, most family therapists will need to be skilled in diagnosing these categories of illness.

Event	Negative Feeling	Negative Thought

FIGURE 5.4. Automatic thoughts journal.

ESTABLISH LONG-TERM TREATMENT GOALS

Now that the therapist has several lenses with which to understand the problems presented by the client, he or she must determine with the family the treatment goals for therapy. The purpose of developing therapeutic goals is multifaceted. In the current managed care climate, goals are often used for accountability—to determine the length of treatment and its effectiveness. Goals tend to be measurable and to describe behavioral changes that are expected, such as specifying an increase or decrease of a problem behavior or symptom. An example could be the decrease of crying spells in a depressed client or the increase in school attendance for the client having a truancy problem. The more vague the goal, the more difficult it will be for you and the client to know whether treatment is progressing.

Workable goals should be stated positively, or in terms of what the client wants to have happen. This is in contrast to the clients' usual pattern of stating problems negatively, outlining what they don't want to happen. One way to help clients focus on a positive statement of goals is to ask a solution-focused question: "What will it look like once the problem is gone?"

Goals assist us in developing a direction for the therapy and a sense of mutuality of purpose. The therapist may offer some suggestions of goals after he or she begins to understand the problem the clients experience and can conceptualize the beginning direction of treatment. Goals need to be elicited from each of the family members and considered by all. At times, goals of outside persons (e.g., school teachers, case workers) tied to the case must be recognized as pertinent also.

Mutual therapeutic goals are acceptable to all family members and to the therapist—that is, everyone agrees these goals are valuable to pursue in therapy. An example is a family presenting with constant arguments and power struggles that culminate in someone being verbally abusive. A mutual goal might be to increase their positive communication and to eliminate the abusive talk. The responsibility for the problem lies with all therapy participants—family and therapist alike.

Also, families often present with multiple problems, and the therapist may choose to use a variety of theoretical perspectives to help them. In the earlier case example about the depressed middle-aged woman, the client presented to the therapist several issues: depression, the husband's alcohol consumption and her increased arguing with him, her changing relationship with her children, and her conflictual relationship with her mother. Each of these areas are legitimate for therapy and might even be conceptualized from different points of view. The therapist, with the client, must determine the order in which these issues would be addressed.

In this case, it was agreed that the client's depression was of first priority. After several sessions and some relief of the depression, the therapist and client might begin to address her relationship with her husband and possibly invite him into therapy. Antidepressant medication may also be started through referral to a physician for medication evaluation.

At times the client's goals may differ from those of the therapist. An angry and frustrated father who is separated may use therapy as evidence that he is a better parent than his wife. This may not be a goal with which the therapist can agree. Mutual goals aid in establishing a collaborative, cooperative therapeutic environment where the process of therapy involves ongoing evaluation. Once goals have been established, the therapist and client will evaluate their progress together. Identifying realistic goals helps us determine what can be accomplished in the course of therapy. Tangible behavioral changes, such as decreasing arguments or quitting consumption of alcohol, can be observed and quantified. Changes in attitude or personal feelings are less tangible and more difficult to measure.

Although the therapist must provide hope for the family that change can happen, it is equally important to be realistic about the limits of therapy. In a summation of some major findings on psychotherapy, Grunebaum (1988) notes that couple and family therapy are helpful for probably about two thirds to three quarters of all clients seen. This indicates that between 25% to 33% of clients will not benefit from our therapy. Nichols (1988) describes one of the contraindications of marital therapy as a couple's refusal or inability to engage in it. For example, extreme hostility and continuous nonproductive communication may make progress in couple therapy impossible. If therapy is going to move beyond support to assist the clients in making changes, there must be some cooperation and motivation to change on the part of the family.

Factors outside therapy, such as socioeconomic issues or a lack of adequate community resources, can impact the client's ability to set treatment goals. A 27-year-old single mother of two children, with a limited education, living in an inner city, must address issues of her economic survival before she is able to consider her own or her family's psychological well-being. The therapist may adapt the therapeutic goals to provide support, information, and resources to this client and assist her in achieving a level of stability rather than seeking to assist her in change.

A client's history and any preexisting psychopathology must be considered in evaluating treatment goals. The family's history in previous treatment is very useful diagnostic and treatment planning information. Too often therapists do not obtain previous history, they find it dated or irrelevant to their therapy. However, information from a previous therapist can help determine what interventions will be more effective and what might be unproductive. Where the family is likely or unlikely to change may become clearer.

SELECT TREATMENT MODALITY, OBJECTIVES, AND INTERVENTIONS

The next step is for the therapist to select the framework and specific theory that might best help address the presenting problem. The selection arises from several interacting factors: the orientation and the experience of the therapist, professional research, financial constraints upon the therapy, a determination of how long therapy should last, and the willingness and availability of family members to participate in the therapeutic experience.

Therapist's Orientation

Early family therapists often identified themselves with one particular school of family therapy. It was common in the 1970s for family therapists to identify themselves with a particular theoretical school, as in "I'm a structural family therapist" or "I'm Bowenian." This was the era when training sites and their leaders were aligned with a particular school of family therapy. A good example is the Philadelphia Child Guidance Clinic, with Salvador Minuchin as its central figure and structural family therapy as its focus. In addition, university training programs frequently taught only one or two theories, often structural and strategic family therapy. Family therapists who trained during this era would usually treat every client they saw using their favorite theoretical orientation. The particular details of the client's situation might be overlooked as the therapist searched for information that fit the theoretical model.

Currently, most family therapists will be trained in a variety of theoretical perspectives. Some will make more sense to you than others, and some of the clinical skills associated with the theories will seem more natural for you to practice than others. Most beginning therapists need to try out several theoretical orientations and their associated skills with clients during their practicum training. Depending on your comfort zone and your training, you will be attracted to particular ways of conceptualizing and treating the problems presented to you by your clients.

It is important to recognize both the strengths and limits of practicing family therapy from your comfort zone. For example, if you believe that past issues influence the present, you might be drawn toward a historical or transgenerational perspective. Understanding and treating the depression experienced by the client in the case example using a genogram and coaching for differentiation might be your first treatment choice. However, transgenerational work might take longer to treat the depression than would other perspectives.

Therapist's Experience

Over time, therapists draw on the wealth of knowledge and experience they have to help their clients (Grunebaum, 1988). Although therapists continue to draw on theory to ground their understanding of the problem, practical clinical experience may provide useful and effective strategies for helping with a specific problem. For example, "scheduling" grieving opportunities for those dealing with loss may be useful even if you don't understand how it works theoretically. Requesting that a couple have a fun date night without discussing their problems may be valuable even if you don't work from a behavioral perspective. Therapists, like any professionals, make use of what works.

Professional Research

Research models inside and outside family therapy may direct us to therapeutic models that can help guide solid clinical work. Some family therapy models provide a clear description of their match with a specific problem and empirical support for their efficacy. Lester Greenberg and Susan Johnson (1988) developed emotionally focused therapy—a blend of systemic, Gestalt, and attachment theories—and offered empirical support for this model for treating distressed couples' relationships. John Gottman (1994) developed a model of minimal marital therapy, which grew out of his 20 years of longitudinal work predicting divorce. A psychoeducational model from Brown University effectively treats patients with manic--depressive disorders and their families. These are just a few examples of research-supported matches between problems and treatment. Family therapists can use research to guide and support their interventions, while maintaining their specific clinical orientation. For example, in the case study on depression, professional research supports the use in therapy of combined medication and cognitive-behavioral techniques to reduce depressive symptoms. Increasingly, treatment guidelines for specific disorders are based on a foundation of research. Authorization and utilization case workers want to know that therapists know and use this information.

Financial Constraints

If your client holds insurance that pays for two to three sessions at 80%, then pays 50% for another six sessions, then nothing, he or she may want to use a "quicker fix" orientation due to these financial concerns. You may feel pressured to use a brief therapy model that focuses on a specific problem with the goal of reducing or eliminating the client's distress. In the case study, solution-focused therapy along with cognitive-behavioral work may decrease some of the client's oppressive symptoms of depression. A referral for medication evaluation may also be made. Underlying issues that may contribute to the cause of the problem, such as family of origin conflicts, may not be adequately addressed within this brief therapy framework. The therapist can negotiate whether or not the client wishes to pay for services beyond what is provided by insurance benefits. Clearly, the impact of managed care on limiting the type and length of mental health services continues to shape our field. Therapists must be able to offer clinically reasonable information as they become more accountable to the payers of their client's benefits.

Client's Willingness and Availability

Each theoretical framework guides the therapist's choice of specific persons to invite into the therapy room. If structural therapy is selected, at least two generations need to be present; if strategic therapy is chosen, whoever is involved in the "stuck cycles of interaction" may be included. In the early days of family therapy, some schools took a strong stand about who should come to therapy: everyone. These early family therapists even suggested that the initial session not be held until the entire family could come. Today most family therapists are less adamant. Involving the client in negotiating the therapy process predicts compliance with treatment recommendations and greater likelihood of a successful outcome. In addition, more recent family therapy approaches have taken a less authoritarian tone and a more constructivist view. The family and the therapist co-create an understanding of the problem, including who is involved and, thus, who should come to therapy. Practicality also comes into play. One or more persons in the family may not be available or willing to take part in treatment on a regular basis. Some family therapy theories require certain people to be in the room for the interventions to be effective. You may not be able to use such a theory and its related interventions with a particular family, based on some of these limitations.

The therapist might also offer options for the client regarding the way therapy will be conducted. This is especially helpful for a family who has been in therapy before. Recently, a couple came in for help with their 11-year-old daughter and reported that they had been in some sort of therapy for about seven years of this child's life. Determining what had already been tried and had worked or failed needed to be discussed before moving into the treatment focus. The parents stated that they had already looked at their own childhoods. They thought that certain behavioral strategies were helpful, but they needed to adapt them to the needs of an older child. They also found themselves at odds with each other, and knew they needed help in working together in their discipline.

Being able to conceptualize the presenting problems from several vantage points will help determine which theoretical framework and interventions make most sense to you. If one theory seems to fit and you have the necessary skills, proceed with treatment. If you understand clearly how a particular theory would address your client's problem, but you have limited experience in using the interventions associated with that theory, rely on supervision and focused self-education to direct you. If you could offer therapy from more than one theoretical perspective, you might discuss the options with the family. In this way, the family can understand the changes they must make, and they will be more willing to engage in the work. Taking into account your own therapy orientation, your experience, professional research, financial constraints, and the client's willingness and availability help you to match interventions that provide the best fit for particular families with particular problems.

DETERMINE LENGTH AND FREQUENCY OF TREATMENT

In the past, most therapists and clients never made an explicit decision about the length of treatment. Treatment started and lasted as long as the clients or the therapist wanted. The therapy might have slowly evolved over time, so even when the presenting problem was resolved, therapy continued as new issues emerged. The historical influence of psychoanalysis, in which therapy was frequent and lasted over several years, probably led most people to think of therapy as at least a yearlong venture.

Except for those who pay independently for mental health services, this is no longer the situation. Concerns about cost and the lack of empirical support for the contention that longer therapy is, in fact, more successful have led to a growing trend toward brief, time-limited treatments. Today, therapy may be time-limited because the payer sets a limit on the number of sessions allowed. Length of therapy is no longer a decision made between the therapist and client, but is strongly influenced by other considerations.

Family therapy has always focused on brief, problem-focused treatments. For some approaches, the average number of sessions is about six. Family therapists focus on a specific problem and when that problem is solved, the therapy ends. When tangential issues arise, they are only addressed in relation to the presenting problem. For example, a client comes in because he feels unable to form a lasting, intimate relationship. During the third session he mentions that he also feels overweight and unable to lose weight. Instead of changing the focus to weight issues, the matter would be addressed only in terms of how it influences the client's initiatives at forming relationships.

Beginning family therapists make two common mistakes regarding the length of therapy. First, even when they have set therapeutic goals, they change the focus each session depending on the "problem of the week." In our program, we begin to identify "problem of the week" families and recognize that therapy with them may go on forever. Another common problem is that the therapist and family meet the stated goal and decide to keep doing therapy anyway. An important skill for a beginning therapist is to know when to end therapy (see Chapter 11 for a detailed discussion of termination). This criterion should be at least partially established when the goals are set. Thus, therapy ends when the goals are met, and goals are set utilizing a realistic timetable.

While insurance companies may play a role in determining length of treatment, clearly it is the client and the nature of the problem that should guide the therapist in deciding the best modality of treatment—either crisis intervention, brief, or long-term treatment. Table 5.3 provides a number of helpful indicators that can be used when making decisions about length of therapy.

Frequency of sessions may range from several times a week, if the family is in severe crisis, to a regular monthly appointment over a period of several months. Clients can also be seen following termination for a follow-up or check-up session. Sessions can be held with greater frequency at the beginning of therapy, weekly for example, and move to every other week as the family progresses and moves toward termination.

Frequency of sessions is determined by practical and logistical issues as well as clinical or treatment concerns. As mentioned earlier, external guidelines may be constructed by an agency, a health maintenance organization, or the client's insurance company, which may set a limit on the number of sessions per week. It is common practice for therapy to be limited to a maximum of two sessions per week with no more than one session on a given day. Time, money, and scheduling factors may also affect session frequency. Coordinating client and therapist schedules can place some limits on available times. In couple and family therapy there tends to be a premium on late afternoon appointments.

The client's need and level of motivation will assist in determining the session frequency. Highly anxious clients may need to come in more frequently at first, in order to work toward their stated goals: More frequent visits allow them to solve problems over a shorter period of time.

Staggering sessions over a longer time, perhaps every second or third week, can be used to determine how changes are being integrated. If the

TABLE 5.3. Length of Therapy Indicators

Indicators for crisis intervention

1. There is a severe disruption in client or family's normal functioning.
2. Client's response to an event is extremely overwhelmed and highly stressed.
3. An external event has occurred suddenly and caused considerable psychological or emotional instability.
4. Family or client has been traumatized by an external event or a developmental change.
5. Client is in danger or harming self or other.
6. Client's symptoms have intensified to the point of causing incapacitation.

Indicators for brief therapy

1. Agency or institutional policy dictates a limited number of visits.
2. Client's goals for therapy are essentially symptom-focused.
3. Client or family is receptive to therapy and willing to change.
4. Client or family has additional resources available to support and integrate change.
5. Clear changes in behavior can be observed.
6. Client's or family's history is not a primary concern.

Indicators for long-term therapy

1. Client's or family's history has significant bearing on presenting concerns.
2. Client or family can engage in a longer-term therapeutic relationship.
3. Client's concerns go beyond behavioral issues and involve underlying dynamics or causes.
4. Client's goals for therapy include identifying and sustaining changes during therapy.
5. There is a significant amount of anxiety and concern that warrants longer-term work.

---

client is seen less frequently, then the therapy may be used to process changes that have occurred and evaluate their impact. In this context, therapy can support and pace changes that have happened between sessions. Periodic meetings can be established after termination on an as-needed basis. Therapy should be viewed as a safe place to return to without the client feeling like a failure. Follow-up sessions should offer a review of progress that has occurred and support for the client's successes.

In addition to determining how often sessions should occur, therapists need to decide how long individual meetings will last. Tradition suggests sessions of 45–50 minutes, or perhaps 90 minutes for a family session. Clearly, most meetings have a beginning, middle, and an end. The therapist needs to pace the session so that the ending is not abrupt, but anticipated. Moving toward a summary with 10 or 15 minutes left to go can be helpful in providing adequate closure.

CONSIDER REFERRALS TO OUTSIDE RESOURCES

The final step in the initial treatment plan asks the therapist to consider if other therapeutic resources might be needed to assist the client.

Knowing the resources available within the community is a necessary part of your responsibilities as a family therapist. Purchasing local directories of clinical services and resources, having some working knowledge of self-help groups, and networking with other professionals who provide expertise in specific areas will be a developing aspect of your work. Agencies often organize this information better than do private practitioners, and it often takes 6 months to a year to have a solid handle on local resources if the community is a large one. Having access to outside resources enables therapists to provide clients with a written list of supplemental contacts they might find helpful. Clients often see this move as enhancing and not detracting from the authority of the therapist.

Referrals to other mental health professionals also might be considered, particularly when there is limited progress in therapy or the therapist feels in over his or her head. Often it's helpful to discuss this feeling with the client, too, allowing the client either to provide reassurances that therapy is working, or to better clarify needs. Beginning therapists think this kind of discussion will undermine their authority; our experience as supervisors indicates the opposite impact. Clients often appreciate the therapist's concern and begin to emphasize what is "working differently" in their relationships, which in turn helps to continue positive clinical work. One warning however—some clients, especially those with abandonment issues, might interpret a discussion about referrals as meaning that you don't want to work with them. For these clients one needs to be particularly careful. Getting supervision will be important before bringing up the topic (see supervisory and peer consultations discussed in Chapter 10).

Finally, an essential quality of a competent therapist working from a biopsychosocial perspective is acknowledgment of the limits of one's particular field of knowledge. During treatment planning especially, therapists are encouraged to consider consultations with other health care professionals. Generally, the success of referrals for both medication or testing consultations depends on the therapist's ability to be clear and concise about what information one hopes to obtain from the referrals. The following sections highlight indications, procedures, and special considerations related to consultations with medical and psychological professionals.

Medication Consultations

Family therapists have been reticent to use psychotropic medications as part of their treatment planning (Patterson & Magulac, 1994). In fact, in the early years of family therapy, using medication could be seen as an admission of failure. Recently, attitudes about using medication have changed. Therapists who do not have a medical degree and thus cannot prescribe medication are becoming open to a joint treatment model wherein they work with a physician (usually a psychiatrist, internist, family physician, or pediatrician) in coordinating treatment. The physician prescribes and manages the psychotropic medication while the therapist provides the "talk therapy."

Family therapists need to make medication referrals with caution. Negative side effects of medication are common. In addition, patients can interpret the referral as the therapist saying "You are really crazy—too crazy for family therapy" or as the therapist abandoning the client to another provider. However, medication should not be overlooked as an option. Frequently, family therapists have no training or knowledge about psychotropic medications and have limited biological knowledge; thus, they do not consider medication as a possible intervention. In addition, therapists fear losing control of their client's treatment or view referral to another provider as a sign of failure or inadequacy. For all these reasons, family therapists might not consider making a medication referral.

While family therapists support the idea of a biopsychosocial model of assessment and treatment, the biological part is rarely emphasized or even considered. However, a true biopsychosocial model would consider both assessment of biological influences, such as genetic history, and biologically based treatment, including medication and surgery. This holistic approach argues for including a biomedical provider if the therapist does not have expertise in biological assessment.

Beyond the biopsychosocial model, other reasons compel therapists to consider medication consultations. One reason is that their clients ask about it. Research in the last 10 years has produced powerful new psychotropic medications, such as Prozac, with fewer negative side effects. Popular articles on the success of these new drugs can be found on any newsstand. Another reason therapists might consider medication is that they work in a setting where the biomedical model is paramount and physicians are in charge. Settings like health maintenance organizations and preferred provider organizations encourage using medication because it is often a relatively inexpensive, effective treatment.

Speed of treatment is another reason therapists consider medication. Timeliness and cost are key criteria in many therapy settings. While it may constitute sloppy treatment, many therapist feel pressure to utilize a "shotgun" approach in which every possible treatment is given to the patient. Since medication can bring rapid symptomatic improvement, there is increasing emphasis on using medication from the start of treatment (Griffith & Griffith, 1994).

Changes within the profession also account for the growing awareness of medication. The early years of family therapy were characterized
by a period of marking boundaries and separating from mainstream traditional mental health treatments. As family therapy has become an established profession, magnifying its distinctions has become less important. Instead of acknowledging only the family as the patient, most family
therapists today will recognize one family member as perhaps needing a
biologically based treatment while the rest of the therapy remains focused
on family interaction. Although family therapists cannot prescribe or
monitor medications, they have an obligation to clients to assess for or
otherwise recognize various problems and pathologies that might benefit
from psychotropic drugs. Knowing when to and how to obtain a psychiatric consultation is an important part of our work, as the following case
demonstrates.

Bill, a 39-year-old man, presented with marital problems including
constant arguing, financial problems, and a lack of mutual interests. Mary
was a 37-year-old woman who had just begun to work full-time as an
insurance sales agent. She complained about Bill's moodiness and lack
of involvement with the family, saying, "All he wants to do is to be left
alone." Bill had worked as a stockbroker for the previous 10 years and
indicated that business had been bad and was taking up more of his time
than usual. This couple was seen in marital therapy for four visits. The
husband quickly identified himself as "the problem," and said he felt an
inability to control the way he felt and his negative attitude. He also
expressed some anger toward his wife for her lack of support, particularly since she had started working full-time. The wife said that she felt
she had been supporting her husband for years and needed to do something for herself. Both indicated that they felt lonely in this relationship
and had little understanding of how things had deteriorated to this point
of dissatisfaction. Further exploration of their individual issues indicated
that the husband displayed several depressive symptoms, including a poor
appetite, an erratic sleep pattern, a lack of energy, and irritability. He
said he had been feeling "down" for the past several years and really
couldn't remember when it seemed to have started. Family history indicated that he felt traumatized and partially responsible for his brother's
accidental death when Bill was 14.

The duration and magnitude of Bill's depressive symptoms indicated
that an evaluation for antidepressant medication was warranted. Since
the marriage was presented as the primary problem, it was to be anticipated that either Bill or his wife might have been reluctant to consider
medication. They didn't come to marital therapy expecting to see a physician in addition to a couple therapist. They both had some preconceived
notions about the uses of psychopharmacological drugs. Some discussion

of their experiences with medications and education about psychotropic drugs were necessary. It was also important for the therapist to present Bill's need for a medication evaluation as being in the couple's best interest. Referrals are most effective if they are presented as beneficial to the client. In this case, Bill was receptive to seeing a psychiatrist for a medical evaluation. His wife's primary concern was that medication was "a crutch and addicting." It was suggested that she see the psychiatrist with her husband in order to find answers to any questions and concerns. Both agreed to go to the initial appointment.

Finally, family therapists cannot ignore the burgeoning research indicating a biological role for at least some mental disorders, such as schizophrenia, bipolar illness, autism, and other diseases thought previously to originate in dysfunctional family patterns. Recognizing a biological etiology naturally leads to a biological treatment, frequently medication.

With increasing public awareness about medication, the family therapist needs to learn more about psychotropic drugs. Perhaps one of the best ways to learn is through on-the-job training—experience is a most powerful influence in demonstrating the efficacy of medication for certain problems. Establishing a professional relationship with a psychiatrist or primary care physician who is willing to use a joint treatment model is an ideal way to learn about medication. If possible, we try to personally know the physician we are sending our patients to for medical evaluations so that we can be sure of both their competence and interpersonal skills. Other possibilities include participating in a continuing education course or reading one of the many books on psychotropic medications for nonphysicians. A brief "primer" on commonly used medications is provided in Table 5.4.

Psychological Testing Consultations

Another consultation possibility is to refer a client for psychological testing, to obtain a more standardized report on observations the therapist has already made or a more in-depth description of some aspect of a client's life. When making a testing referral, the therapist should be as specific as possible about what he or she would like to learn. Therapists should be familiar with the variety of tests available and know what to ask for. Whereas one would use a physician for a medication consultation, psychologists are the mental health professionals with specialty training in tests and measures. Usually a report is written based on the tests the psychologist administers. Major types of tests include intelligence tests, projective tests, self-report instruments that describe some aspect of the client's emotional life, and behavioral checklists that describe behavior.

Testing is most commonly used in psychiatric hospitals, school settings, forensic work, and other institutional settings where standardized

TABLE 5.4. Psychotropic Drug Primer

Drugs for anxiety

Benzodiazepines	Includes diazepam (Valium), chlordiazepoxide (Librium), alprazolam (Xanax), clorazepate (Tranxene), halazepam (Paxipam), lorazepam (Ativan), oxazepam (Serax), and prazepam (Centrax).
Buspirone	BuSpar, a nonbenzodiazepine antianxiety drug, does not cause sedation or functional impairment, or have high potential for abuse. Takes 1–2 weeks for effect.
Tricyclics and MAO inhibitors	Tricyclic antidepressants or monoamine oxidase (MAO) inhibitors can prevent panic attacks. Alprazolam is also effective.
Propranolol	Inderal and other beta-blockers are useful in preventing performance anxiety or "stage fright" by suppressing peripheral autonomic symptoms of anxiety.
Adverse effects	Undesirable degree of sedation, anterograde amnesia, dependence (with chronic use), withdrawal (gradual tapering is important), rebound anxiety. Potentially dangerous if taken with other central nervous system depressants (e.g., alcohol, barbiturates).

Drugs for depression

Tricyclics and newer antidepressants	Major tricyclics include imipramine (Tofranil) and amitriptyline (Elavil). Newer antidepressants include amoxapine (Asendin), maprotiline (Ludiomil), trazodone (Desyrel), and fluoxetine (Prozac). Tricyclic treatment failure is often caused by inadequate dosage, insufficient duration of treatment, and poor compliance. Monitoring is critical. Bipolar depression is usually treated with lithium; if depression develops, an antidepressant may be added. Treatment of bipolar depression with an antidepressant alone may trigger a manic episode.
MAO inhibitors	Phenelzine (Nardil) or tranylcypromine (Parnate) is used for patients who can't tolerate or don't respond to tricyclics. Subtypes of depression may benefit from these. Severe depression with psychotic symptoms may require antipsychotic drugs with an antidepressant.
ECT	Electroconvulsive therapy (ECT) has been used for depression that is resistant to antidepressants and may be superior for severely depressed patients, those with delusions or psychomotor retardation, suicidal patients, and some elderly patients.
Adverse effects	Tricyclics: anticholinergic effects, orthostatic hypotension, sedation, weight gain, withdrawal symptoms. Overdosage can be lethal (reactions include cardiac arrhythmias, hypotension, convulsions, and coma). MAO inhibitors: hypertensive reactions.

(cont.)

TABLE 5.4. (cont.)

Drugs for mania

Lithium	Lithium (Eskalith and others) is used for long-term mainte-nance to prevent depressive and manic episodes in bipolar disorder. Because lithium takes 2–3 weeks to have an effect, acutely manic patients may be treated temporarily with antipsychotic drugs such as chlorpromazine (Thorazine) or haloperidol (Haldol). During depressive episodes, a tricyclic or MAO inhibitor may be used in addition to lithium.
Adverse effects	Nausea and fatigue in first weeks of treatment; tremor, thirst, polyuria, edema, weight gain may persist throughout treatment; confusion and ataxia are toxic effects that may not be perceived as drug induced; skin reactions (acne, psoriasis); cardiac and other birth defects. Patients on lithium should avoid pregnancy and should not breastfeed infants.

Drugs for obsessive–compulsive disorder

Antidepressants	Some antidepressants may be used for symptom relief. Clomipramine (Anafranil) is under investigation. Fluoxetine (Prozac) may also be helpful.

Drugs for psychoses

Phenothiazines	A broad class of antipsychotic drugs include such medica-tions as chlorpromazine (Thorazine), fluphenazine (Prolixin), mesoridazine (Serentil), perphenazine (Trilafon), piperacetazine (Quide), prochlorperazine (Compazine), promazine (Sparine), thioridazine (Mellaril), trifluoperazine (Stelazine), and triflupromazine (Vesprin). Symptoms of acute psychosis may improve rapidly after treatment with antipsychotic drugs, but chronic schizophrenia requires 3 or more weeks before a benefit is seen and full improvement may take months. Many chronic patients require prolonged maintenance therapy, but the benefits may be limited and the risk of tardive dyskinesia is considerable.
Adverse effects	Anticholinergic effects (dry mouth, constipation, etc.), drowsiness, postural hypotension, extrapyramidal effects (rigidity, akinesia, tremor), tardive dyskinesia (involuntary movements of lips, tongue, fingers, toes, or trunk) among the frequent or occasional effects of antipsychotic drugs.

Drugs for organic mental syndromes

Antipsychotic drugs	"Organic mental syndromes" refers to mental disorders in which the etiology is either a general medical condition, a substance, or a combination of these (e.g., dementia, delirium, withdrawal). Specific treatments are generally used when treating these disorders, but occasionally small doses of antipsychotic drugs are used to treat symptoms (e.g., perphenazine, fluphenazine, or haloperidol).

(cont.)

TABLE 5.4. (cont.)

Drugs for organic mental syndromes	
Adverse effects	Common side effects are noted under the section titled "Drugs for Psychoses." Benzodiazepines and other sedatives are used with caution for patients with organic mental syndromes because they decrease the ability of patients to perform personal tasks, which may already be marginal, and can aggravate mental confusion.

Note. Adapted from *The Medical Letter* (1991, pp. 43–50). Copyright 1991 by *The Medical Letter.* Adapted by permission.

information beyond the therapist's clinical observations is sought. For example, parents and teachers may request testing when they have a concern about a child's behaviors or abilities. Legal experts may request testing when they are concerned about their client's mental stability or cognitive capacities. A typical psychological report would include the following information: reason for testing and referral source, brief history and description of the client, tests administered, test results, and recommendations.

When would a family therapist ask for psychological testing? Besides the legal and academic reasons just mentioned, the therapist might consider testing in the following situations:

1. A client is not processing information or following the conversation (i.e., signs of possible cognitive problems).
2. The client displays aberrant, inappropriate behavior.
3. A mental status exam reveals problems.
4. A client show signs of a major mental disorder.
5. Corroborative information is needed for legal purposes.
6. A student is referred to therapy for learning, emotional, and/or behavioral problems.

There are also reasons not to do testing. Clients can experience psychological testing as intrusive and tedious, or they may see little reason to participate. Referral to a consultant also brings in another professional and an additional therapeutic relationship. The therapist or the client may be concerned about privacy and confidentiality, and want as little formal documentation as possible. Psychological testing can be expensive, and clients or third party payers may be reluctant to bear the added expense.

If testing is done, the family therapist, the clients, and the recommending agency frequently find the results to be helpful, but this is not always the case. Family therapists need basic tools to evaluate the quality of the report. Probably the most common criticism of test results is that they are too vague or abstract. Having read the results, the therapist might respond "So what?" The report will have value when it offers information pertinent to the direction of treatment.

To improve the chances of receiving a relevant report, a family therapist can become familiar with what tests are available and the qualities of a good report. One way to identify a helpful test is to take some (e.g., the Minnesota Multiphasic Personality Inventory [MMPI] or a family therapy instrument like the Dyadic Adjustment Scale) and consider whether or not the information is useful. Another helpful thing to do is to read a number of testing reports; quality reports will stand out. Family therapists frequently learn about two or three psychologists in their community who do excellent evaluations of children, mental functioning, or other areas. Asking these examiners to do evaluations of some of the therapist's own clients will begin the collaborative relationship.

CONCLUSION

Developing a treatment focus allows the beginning therapist to move from being a good listener to becoming a professional. By using an initial treatment plan, you will be able to conceptualize and explain how therapy will address the painful presenting problems brought to you. Suggestions on who needs to be in therapy, how long the therapy may last, and what methods you will use can be articulated and offered to the family as well as to managed care concerns. Networking with other professionals or community groups may also benefit clinical care. Table 5.5 illustrates what an initial treatment plan might look like using the four family therapy frameworks discussed in this chapter. Having optional ways to address the same presenting problems also helps therapists find a comfortable fit for themselves and the family's they serve.

TABLE 5.5. Initial Treatment Plans

Historical framework

Step 1:	Depression
Step 2:	History of depressive episodes; no previous therapy
Step 3:	Major Depressive Episode, Recurrent (DSM-IV 296.23)
Step 4:	Understand impact of depressive patterns from family of origin; increase differentiation
Step 5:	Transgenerational theory; individual therapy; generate genogram; coach differentiation regarding gender patterns; process grief
Step 6:	12–15 sessions; weekly sessions
Step 7:	Referral for medication evaluation

(cont.)

TABLE 5.5. (cont.)

Structural framework

Step 1: Depression

Step 2: History of depressive episodes; no previous therapy; consultation with MD but no medications taken

Step 3: Major Depressive Episode, Recurrent (DSM-IV 296.23)

Step 4: Solidify couple subsystem; increase husband authority and adult functioning

Step 5: Structural therapy; conjoint sessions with husband and wife; encourage husband to assist wife with housework; assign dates for couple; explore mutual responsibilities for financial support and budgeting; limit telephone contact with mother

Step 6: 8–12 sessions; weekly, then bimonthly

Step 7: Referral for medication evaluation

Process framework

Step 1: Depression

Step 2: History of depressive episodes; no previous therapy; consultation with MD but no medications taken

Step 3: Major Depressive Episode, Recurrent (DSM-IV 296.23)

Step 4: Increase positive communication skills and couple problem solving

Step 5: Strategic and solution-focused therapy; couple therapy; identify negative interactional sequences; explore exceptions of positive communication sequences; use miracle questions to explore future problem solving

Step 6: 6–10 sessions; weekly, then bimonthly

Step 7: Referral for medication evaluation

Experiential framework

Step 1: Depression

Step 2: History of depressive episodes; no previous therapy; consultation with MD but no medication taken

Step 3: Major Depressive Episode, Recurrent (DSM-IV 296.23)

Step 4: Increase affective range and communication between family members

Step 5: Experiential therapy; any combination of family members; identify, explore, and model expression of feelings; validate each family member's affect; use drawings, sculpting, or games to encourage affective expression

Step 6: 10–15 sessions; weekly, then bimonthly

Step 7: Referral for medication evaluation

6

Basic Treatment Skills

K̲aren and Rick stare at each other in frustration. Karen begins, "You don't help with the kids. I can't even. . . ." Rick interrupts, "You're so sensitive. What about the time I took the kids all afternoon . . . ?" Karen rolls her eyes. Sammy, age 9, interrupts, "Don't yell. I can't stand it when you yell." There is an awkward silence in the therapy room.

What skills are necessary to be an effective therapist with a family like this? In this chapter, we first review the elements crucial to relating to your clients. Effective therapists display common qualities no matter what theory or intervention they use. Next, we discuss some basic counseling skills that are the foundation of solid therapeutic work. Finally, marriage and family therapists hold a unique repertoire of skills related to their theoretical perspective. These skills need to be selected intentionally, several guidelines will be offered emphasizing the therapist's role and responsibility in this selection.

THE RUSH TO INTERVENTION VERSUS
DEVELOPING A RELATIONSHIP

Research on the effectiveness of therapy has identified one variable as critical in predicting a positive outcome. While therapists focus on compelling theoretical models or powerful techniques, research suggests that the therapist–client relationship is the most important variable, and, more specifically, the client's perception of the therapist and the relationship

(Grunebaum, 1988). Acknowledging the powerful impact of the therapeutic relationship is both a sobering and humbling experience.

Beginning family therapists who are overwhelmed by their clients' problems and their own sense of inadequacy are often impatient to "do something" in the therapy session. Family therapy students are especially vulnerable to the "do-something syndrome" because their training has usually involved watching numerous master therapists perform brilliant therapeutic techniques on videos. After watching several of these videos and listening to the success of their classmates, students are left wondering why nothing dramatic is happening in their sessions, and the pressure for something to happen intensifies.

This "do-something syndrome" is unfortunate because students fail to recognize their most powerful therapeutic tool—themselves. Often in supervision, we suggest that students sit back, relax, and simply try to get to know and understand the client and his or her story. The point is that before technique and theory can be effective, there must be a relationship. Building it is the first and perhaps central task of the therapy, even for therapists who use a model in which the therapeutic relationship is not a focus.

Showing interest and communicating real empathy are examples of how beginning therapists can use themselves effectively in therapy and begin to build a relationship. Empathy—the ability to enter into a client's subjective world and to utilize one's own life experiences, thoughts, and feelings in relating to the client's pain—creates a powerful bond between the therapist and client and often builds an intimate relationship. Because of this profound connection, therapists must take the responsibility to conduct themselves appropriately with their clients. They need not "take on" the experience of their client to be empathic. The pain belongs to the client, not the therapist. The therapist shares the burden in relieving the difficulties, not in carrying them.

In our experience, there is also some truth to the idea of "fit" between client and therapist. Some therapists will be a good match with particular clients and some will not. A strong lack of fit might signal the therapist to offer a referral to someone else, or to suggest that the client shop for another therapist. In either case, the capacity of the therapist to empathize with the client is a relational quality basic to building the therapeutic alliance.

When one is working with a couple or family, empathy becomes more complicated. The therapist may relate strongly to one member and not to another. These emotional dynamics affect the connections within the clinical session and can be positive or negative contributors to treatment.

Allowing for a variety of empathic attachments within the clinical relationship emotionally taxes the therapist. Beginning family therapists often experience "combat fatigue" during their early work. Some interns think that separating family members and seeing them individually will help the family, but this strategy is actually just self-protective of one's emotional energy. Learning how to create appropriate emotional boundaries with a client is essential for solid work. The ability to stay outside the system while maintaining some emotional attachment to its members is a delicate balancing act for the therapist. Supervision can provide feedback about this balancing, including a number of signs that indicate lack of it, such as going over the session time limit, responding to frequent client phone calls without setting clearer and more stringent guidelines for crisis calls, becoming preoccupied by the client so much that it interferes with other areas of life (insomnia, or thinking about a client all the time), or feeling like you're the only one who can help the client (the savior complex).

Good therapists provide a nonthreatening and trusting climate in which their clients are invited to be honest and to change. Therapists need to communicate a warm and accepting stance even in the midst of looking directly at difficult problems that are impacting clients. For example, a client may warily watch his therapist's reaction when he discloses that he believes his mother may have molested him when he was a child. Ready for blaming or shaming reactions, clients closely monitor how trustworthy and safe the therapist will be.

Trust is primary. Clients often have been accused of being "bad" or "wrong" for feeling, thinking or acting in certain ways. A basic and open acceptance of each person must be in place in order to develop a therapeutic alliance. Clients need to experience the therapist as coming alongside of them and assisting them, not recoiling from them.

Clients also need to know that the therapist will be honest and appropriately self-disclosing when needed. For example, if the therapist is functioning outside of his or her comfort zone about a particular issue, sometimes it may be necessary to let the client know this. Beginning marriage and family therapists often feel this way when they start to provide therapy. Rather than "faking it," being clear about one's status as a trainee, about being supervised, and about working as a team with the client can engender more trust. Of course, trainees need to remember that they, too, have training and expertise from their education, previous clinical exposure, and own life experience to offer to the therapeutic relationship.

As in assessment, curiosity contributes to developing a positive relationship with clients. Especially when working with persons with different life experiences than one's own—whether that difference is related to age or culture, for example—taking a learning posture will often be helpful. It is difficult to stereotype when one takes this position, as a case example illustrates. A Laotian family came into therapy because their

12-year-old had "run away," that is, stayed overnight with a friend her parents didn't know, without telling them. One of the authors asked the parents how 12-year-olds could spend time with their friends in Laos when they were growing up since the therapist didn't know their culture very well. They commented that 12-year-olds spend time with their friends only at school and spend time only with their families outside of school. Families would also get together with other families, and then their children would play together. The therapist asked these parents if they had discussed any "legitimate" way for their daughter to spend time with her peers other than at school or at their home. After looking at each other, they answered that they had not. The daughter then shyly commented that sneaking out was the only way she could be with her friends. The therapist and family then created some new ways for the 12-year-old to spend time with friends (besides school and family gatherings) that the parents and adolescent could accept. Continuing to listen and being curious about your clients' stories doesn't end after the first session. Probing to elicit information about them and their perspectives will promote a safe, healing context for understanding and change.

BASIC COUNSELING SKILLS

The following section highlights several core skills useful for family therapists, although not unique to our profession; they encompass skills utilized by many types of psychotherapies.

Using Questions

From the first phone call, the therapist must use intelligent questions in order to discover needed clinical information. Especially in the early and middle parts of the therapeutic relationship, questions keep the therapy focused upon the client's perceptions and needs. In an effort to clarify the kinds of questions that can be used and the impact of specific types, Tomm (1988) reviews four categories of questions used in uncovering and understanding possibilities for treatment. All questions are seen as having a purpose, an intent, on the part of the therapist.

Figure 6.1 denotes four types of questions based upon particular assumptions deriving from the answers to the following two questions:

1. For whom will the information be used—for the therapist who needs to understand, or for the client who needs to be influenced to change? A continuum extending from "orienting intent" (for the therapist) to "influencing intent" (for the client) may be developed.

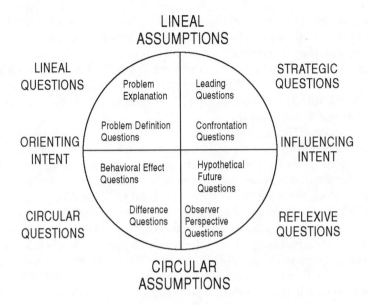

FIGURE 6.1. Question grid. From Tomm (1988, p. 12). Copyright 1988 by *Family Process*. Reprinted by permission.

2. Does therapeutic change occur using linear or circular information? Some kinds of therapy rely more on cause-and-effect information or linear thinking, whereas others rely more on cybernetic or circular information. Family therapy is known for its emphasis on interactional principles and tends to pay more attention to circular questioning in order to gather information. A continuum extending from "lineal assumptions" and "circular assumptions" is developed.

Based on this grid, four kinds of therapist questions can be characterized: lineal, circular, strategic, and reflexive. *Lineal questions* are investigative, deductive, and content-loaded, involving a "just the facts, ma'am" perspective. Information gathered by these questions is thought to explain the problem. For example, questioning about why a child is truant and coming home late may be answered with "He doesn't like it; he hates the teachers; he hates the kids; he didn't like school last year, either; he needs an attitude adjustment." Often lineal questions point to something or someone who is "wrong" and needs to be fixed.

Circular questions are exploratory and stem from a posture of curiosity on the therapist's part. Instead of singling out who or what needs changing, information from these questions highlights interconnections within the family and to larger systems. Underlying the question is the assumption that everything is connected to everything else. A therapist might ask, "What, if anything, is different about the days when your son doesn't cut school?" or "Who in the family first finds out that your son has cut school? What happens after?" Circular questions help to expose patterns in the relationships.

O'Brian and Bruggen (1985) have classified circular questions into four different categories. One type of question has a family member comment on the relationship or interaction between two other family members. For example, the therapist may ask the mother, "How do your son and husband get along?" Or the therapist may ask a child, "What does your mother do when your father comes home and has been drinking?" Another type of circular question may have individuals rank-order family members' responses to an actual or hypothetical situation. A therapist might ask, "Who is most upset about the divorce? Who next?" Or he might ask more generally, "Who will be most relieved when this problem is resolved? Who will be next most relieved?" A third type examines differences that occur over time. Questions can relate to a specific event that happened in the past or is anticipated to happen in the future. For example, a mother might be asked how her child's behavior has changed since the divorce, or a father might be asked how his marriage will change once the children leave home. A fourth type of circular question is used to solicit information indirectly about an individual who is unwilling to answer questions or is not present. A wife may be asked by the therapist, "If your husband were here today, what would he say are the biggest problems in your marriage?"

Circular questions within each category can focus on present, past, or future/hypothetical events. The therapist should not feel restricted to developing circular questions that perfectly fit a classification system. Rather, the different categories highlight a variety of purposes and ways of constructing circular questions, which can stimulate the therapist's creativity. However they are posed, circular questions tease out interconnections between people and behaviors, revealing interacting factors that influence the presenting problem. With this information the therapist can better understand current symptom-maintaining sequences and can develop strategies or explore ways in which these sequences can be disrupted.

A third category on the question grid presented in Figure 6.1 consists of *strategic questions,* or influencing questions, which are challenging in nature. They pose new possibilities, often in a particular direction. A therapist might ask, for example, "What would it take to have you and your ex-husband take a united parental stand with your child on this matter?" or "What might happen if you and your child's father ignored your child's behavior of leaving school early for a few weeks?" In both questions the therapist attempts to interrupt the current interactional sequence by having the parents align their behavioral reactions to their child. The question is purposive and often corrective. Changing the way the family currently responds to a problem is primary when asking strategic questions.

Reflexive questions facilitate change in the family without moving the family in any particular direction. Therapists, through their questions, attempt to mobilize new response possibilities from the family. The therapist assumes clients have and can access internal resources for change. Examples of reflexive questions are "What if your son had some strong feelings that he couldn't share with you, how could you let him know that you wanted to hear them?" or "If your son started attending school regularly again, how would your lives be different?" In both examples, a fairly neutral stance is taken by the therapist, in the belief that the client can find new responses that are "different and better" than previous responses. Rather than focusing on any precise behavior change, the door is opened to alternatives. Reflexive questions facilitate change without directing it.

In all these types of questions, nonverbal as well as verbal skills communicate the posture and perspective of the therapist. For example, a question like "What is your reaction?" can be asked in a demanding or a requesting way. Keeping nonverbal communication and verbal questions congruent allows more effective communication. In any case, the skill of questioning contributes to our ability to act as agents of change in the lives of the families we serve.

Normalizing

Normalizing requires some knowledge of what's normal. It means that the therapist understands the symptoms presented by a client as part of normative behavior connected with particular developmental phases in an individual's or a family's life. Relating a 14–year-old's moody and more private behavioral changes to "a common part of adolescence" often helps relieve a family's concern. Normalizing a couple's distress over decreasing romantic interest while they have two preschool-age children can help them accept and understand rather than fear the changes in their relationship. Often a therapist notices an immediate calming in the client system when something has been normalized. Sometimes the family will respond by offering up stories that validate the normality of the symptoms (for example, when Uncle John had the same problem).

Providing psychoeducational resources such as developmentally sensitive books or self-help groups and readings can be quite helpful for normalizing problems. We have included in this text discussions about normative reactions to life cycle and other developmental issues. Self-help groups also provide a strong normalizing experience for clients, especially those who are more socially isolated. For some, committing to a very short-term treatment contract (three to five sessions) helps to reassure the family that their concerns are interpreted as normal, and sets the appropriate clinical tone for the family. After brief therapy, one can reevaluate if the problem has been adequately addressed after labeling symptoms as normal. Many good developmental texts are available to clinicians to assist in normalizing.

Reframing

Sometimes change can occur through cognitive shifts rather than behavioral shifts. Reframing relies on the therapist's creative ability to reinterpret symptoms presented in therapy. Normalizing is one type of reframing since it attempts to decrease the anxiety about a particular problem by viewing it as normal.

Reframing allows clients to see their issues from another point of view, thus opening up the possibility of new responses. For example, a single mother comes into counseling because of the temper tantrums displayed by her 6-year-old daughter. The mother views this behavior as "willful disobedience and attempting to get her own way." Upon review of the circumstances often accompanying the tantrums, the therapist notes that the child gets very little undivided attention from her mother and then reframes the child's tantrum as a desire to "get more attention from Mom" and a "crying out since she feels lonely inside." Reframing the child's behavior in this way may change the ways the mother responds to her child. New ways the child might receive support from her mother can be considered.

Providing Support

As our society becomes more and more transient, providing a stable, consistent, and nurturing relationship in a client's life often resembles throwing a life jacket to a drowning person. The key way that therapists provide this nurturance is through attentive and active listening to the client's story. As the therapist begins to reflect back, understand, and grant permission to explore any and all feelings or thoughts, clients experience reassurance, a solid foundation from which to build new possibilities. "Just being there" makes a difference.

Yet support, however valuable, does not guarantee change. With the sweeping influence of managed care and the need to justify each dollar spent on mental health care, supportive psychotherapy appears to be in question—almost a luxury. Support is more stabilizing in function than change inducing. Providing a reassuring place to be might not address the problem presented by the client. It must be remembered that clients usually don't seek therapy when everything is great, but rather when they are experiencing pain. This pain signals something significant and must be respected. Support can help to alleviate some of the pain, but often won't remedy it. Change using a supportive stance can be dramatic but often takes a long-term relationship, perhaps 1 or 2 years, before results are seen.

If you wish to explore some of the theoretical ideas behind a supportive posture in therapy, readings in both the self psychology and person-centered literature will be valuable. We recommend *Treating the Self* (Wolf, 1988) and *On Becoming a Person* (Rogers, 1972).

Confronting

To facilitate change, at some point during the therapy clinicians need to ask clients if they really want to change. This may or may not be done directly. Some therapies based on strategic models do not spend much time providing verbal support (although they do provide nonverbal support) and jump right into the domain of confrontation by using strategic or reflexive questions. For example, the first question from a solution-focused therapist might be "What would need to happen during our first session today to help with the problem you called about?" A change posture is expected and clients will be "fired" from therapy if they are unable to respond to change-oriented probing. Confrontation, although delivered with sensitive and concerned words, may begin immediately.

For some therapists and some clients, beginning therapy with a more confrontive posture won't be fitting. These therapists and clients must discover the appropriate time to move into more change-focused activities. Of course, this might be done sooner than one thinks. For example, as soon as a therapist develops an intelligent treatment plan, he or she necessarily moves into the confrontive domain since the treatment plan identifies specific areas to change. Likewise, as soon as the therapist wonders if involving other family members might help the situation, he or she is confronting the status quo. When a therapist tries to evaluate if therapy is helping, he or she moves into doing something different. Confrontation is essential to change.

Systemically oriented therapists know something about the difficulty we have in facilitating change. We know that clients tend to maintain homeostasis—the familiar way of handling a problem. Change takes energy and is often difficult to achieve. Directly or indirectly, the therapist must confront old ways of doing things and seek new possibilities in order for change to occur.

Pacing

The pace at which a therapy session moves involves how slowly or rapidly material is revealed by the client. The therapist's interventions can alter the pace by creating opportunities for further exploration of a particular issue, changing the focus to another topic, adding depth or breadth to the discussion, or exploring the emotions related to the issue. All of these interventions will impact what clients reveal and will lead them in a particular direction. Most interventions will be focused on either pacing or leading the client or family. In its simplest form, pacing involves "following the client." Mirroring a client's behavior enables the therapist to move at the client's pace. Techniques such a reflecting, active listening, and tracking also provide useful vehicles for pacing. Pacing a client is an essential aspect of the joining process and is critical in developing rapport and building a trustful working relationship.

Leading is an attempt by the therapist to select a direction for exploration and lead the client there. Joining with the client must precede moving to a leading stance. If a young man is talking about his concerns about going to college, the therapist might first pace the client's concerns by listening to him. The therapist can then lead him by asking questions about his feelings about college and his thoughts about his ability to be successful. The introduction of the new focus expands the breadth and depth of the discussion and leads the client in a particular direction.

The therapist should monitor the pace of the session. If too much material is revealed too rapidly, there might not be sufficient time to follow up on critical events or issues, or the family's emotional response to a particular concern may be obscured. Slowing down the pace of the session often proves helpful in allowing clients to follow their own belief or feeling about an issue. If the pace is too slow, clients or therapist can become complacent and bored with the session. The therapist may need to intervene to move the session along by asking thought-provoking questions or focusing on present, "here-and-now," behavior. Most sessions will alternate between some pacing of the concerns and some leading to assist in developing alternative directions to be explored.

Several factors should be considered in determining the pace of therapy. If the family is highly motivated to change, then the pace of the therapy can be more rapid. High levels of resistance will likely mean that the pace will be slower. The length of treatment is also a factor. Brief therapy may limit the depth of exploration. The client's level of anxiety will also be a consideration in developing the pace. If anxiety is high the therapist may need to slow things down to assist in containing the client's fears. If the client's anxiety is extremely low there may be a lack of motivation to change, and the pace may need to be increased.

Specific techniques that hasten the pace of therapy include asking open-ended questions, leading in a particular direction, identifying the process in the session, and focusing on the "here and now." Techniques that slow down the pace include tracking and obtaining clarification, mirroring behavior, active listening, and reflecting.

Dealing with Crises

Sometimes therapy begins with a crisis, a situation made up of unique circumstances that tend to be short-term, overwhelming, and understandable in terms of the client's reaction to stress. Sudden and unexpected external events such as the death of a family member, an automobile accident, or a natural disaster are examples of incidents that could cause a client to be under severe stress or "in crisis." Crisis can also occur around developmental or maturational issues such as the birth of a child, a child reaching adolescence, or the last child leaving home. Each individual or family will react to the situation differently and will cope with it idiosyncratically. The crisis state is characterized by severe disruption in the client or family's normal level of functioning. Common symptoms include physical and psychological agitation, poor appetite, loss of sleep, emotional distress, anxiety, and an inability to solve problems. Although the objective reality of a crisis such as a natural disaster may be the same to most people, responses to the event are highly subjective. A client's level of vulnerability will depend upon a subjective interpretation of the event, available resources, and previous history in coping with stress.

Even within a family each person will respond to the crisis differently, which can exacerbate family difficulties. For example, a family was about to go to court to settle an automobile accident in which their 17-year-old son was at fault. The event was causing a severe amount of stress for the parents who had an exhaustive argument prior to the court appearance in which the both became very caustic and verbally abusive. The potential financial threat to their already unstable financial picture caused considerable fear and insecurity. The parents' response to the upcoming court hearing was to become agitated and conflictual, while the young man's response was to withdraw and deny the importance of the problem. Their reactions caused further difficulties between the family members, and, thus, a situational crisis ensued.

Families respond in their characteristic ways to a potential crisis. A crisis may escalate very quickly in a family in which anticipation of a worst-case scenario adds to the problem. In another family a crisis can be avoided through their use of effective problem-solving skills. The family's ability to respond to the crisis will depend on their ability to handle stress and conflict.

Crisis intervention tends to be short-term and present focused. The therapist typically needs to assume an active and directive role in assisting clients when they are under severe stress. Rappaport (1970) has identified four goals for crisis intervention:

1. Relieving the client's immediate symptoms.
2. Restoring the client to his or her previous level of functioning.
3. Identifying the factors that led to the crisis state.
4. Identifying and applying remedial measures.

Crisis intervention techniques will vary, depending on the client's state and the nature of the crisis. Affective interventions will focus on assisting the family in expressing their feelings about the situation as oftentimes there is little opportunity to do so during the actual event. A debriefing period should include expressing feelings and providing support for what the family has been through. Normalizing their response to the situation may also be helpful. Cognitive interventions may focus on altering negative beliefs, guilt, or self-incriminating thoughts. For example, if a family is involved in an accident in which one member dies and another lives, assisting the surviving member in alleviating guilt may be an important initial intervention. Behavioral tasks can assist the client in doing something or taking some action in order to begin to regain a sense of control over life. Beginning to rebuild shortly after a disaster can prove helpful in coping with psychological and material losses. Assisting the family in utilizing community resources from agencies, churches, synagogues, or social programs may also be valuable.

Offering Psychoeducational Information

Another basic resource that can be developed by therapists is verbal and written information that can be provided to family members about common presenting problems. Develop a "handout file" for clients on common issues such as "Communication Skills," "Attention-Deficit/Hyperactivity Disorder," "Depression," "Helping Your Adolescent," "Basics in Parenting," or "Alcoholism," or compile a book list of useful self-help books on various topics can also augment the therapy. The division between academic information and self-help references has become blurred in recent years; therefore, many wonderful books or articles are available for use with families identified with particular life issues.

THE DEVELOPMENT OF EXPERTISE
AS A FAMILY THERAPIST

The relational and systemic perspective of family therapists contributes a unique perspective to change. Competency in the related skills comes with practice. Expertise can be developed by establishing a solid knowledge base, by becoming more sophisticated in using interventions, by knowing your role in therapy, and by creating treatment plans from a family therapy perspective.

Establish a Solid Knowledge Base

Most family therapy interventions can be clearly derived from a theoretical explanation of why change occurs. Thus, your treatment skills need to develop from a solid understanding of their theoretical foundation. For example, structural family therapy holds that the problems presented by a family stem from faulty family structure, usually inappropriate hierarchy (e.g., the children holding the power in the family) and/or inappropriate boundaries (e.g., family members disengaged or isolated). In order to help the family with its presenting problem, the therapist must be able to use the "tools," or interventions, associated with the theory about the problem. For example, a structural therapist might begin by requesting an "enactment" (structural intervention 1) of the fight the mother and daughter were just talking about during the therapy session. The therapist asks the mother and daughter to "show me and let me listen in on" the fight they had on Friday night. After the therapist observes the "fight" for awhile (mentally developing a structural map of the family relationships; structural intervention 2), he or she may intervene by asking the mother to stop the conversation with her daughter and turn toward her husband and discuss her concerns with him. In this way the therapist has intervened to "realign the parental subsystem" (structural intervention 3), since the father had previously been underinvolved. A structural therapist needs to understand why and how change might be accomplished for a client using structural tools. He or she must know when and how to apply the interventions are associated with the theory, with that conceptualization of change.

Each family therapy theory entails several specific interventions that can lead to change. In order to intervene skillfully, you must be clear about what theoretical stance you are using and the skills associated with that stance. There are several wonderful texts that explain each family therapy theory and their related interventions. Excellent overview texts are *Family Therapy: Concepts and Methods* (Nichols & Schwartz, 1991), *Handbook of Family Therapy* (Gurman & Kniskern, 1991), and, for couples, *Clinical Handbook of Couple Therapy* (Jacobson & Gurman, 1995). After you have learned about the theory and have tried out the interventions with actual families, you will need to develop the skills at more sophisticated levels, intermediate and, ultimately, advanced.

Probably the best way to develop your interventions is to attend all-day or weekend skill-based workshops. Learning about and actually practicing interventions associated with transgenerational, structural, narrative, solution-focused, emotionally focused, cognitive-behavioral, or object relations theory by presenters who train and specialize in these areas will be extremely useful. Purchasing books written for clinicians within a particular theoretical focus can help too. You can further improve your competency within a particular theoretical focus by being supervised by a person who works from that particular perspective. As you move to other internships or work settings, you can deliberately aim to work with clinicians who are proficient in a specific school of clinical work.

Besides being clear about your theoretical grounding, specializing in the treatment of a distinctive population can be useful. For example, treating domestic violence, eating disorders, substance abuse, or sexual problems, or doing divorce mediation can be specialized work. Information on the characteristics of each group, researched and effective treatment strategies (often integrating several therapeutic disciplines), and guidelines for early–middle–later stages of therapy may be available to assist you in working with these families. You don't always have to hypothesize what will be helpful; others may have acquired useful information you can now incorporate in your work. Again, workshops, books, and supervisors with expertise are wonderful resources to help in the development of your intervention skills.

Become More Sophisticated in Using Interventions

In addition to choosing a theoretical framework from which to do therapy and possibly specializing in a specific population, therapists must consider issues of process and content, timing, and even clients' anxiety levels when selecting specific interventions.

O'Hanlon (1982) has identified 13 classes of intervention that delineate different options for intervening in personal and interpersonal patterns of behavior, perception, and experience. These interventions are focused on altering patterns of behavior as they affect symptoms. For example, if the family presents constant arguing as the problem, the intervention is used to disrupt the pattern by altering how often arguments take place.

Interventions can focus on the process or content of a dialogue or interaction. The content of an interaction is what is actually said, while the process is how it is said (Satir, 1967). For example, a father and his 15-year-old son might be discussing the young man's desire to get his driver's license. This issue is the content of *what* is being discussed. The process, or *how* it is being discussed, includes underlying feelings of concern, the tone of the discussion, and the communication pattern. Interventions that focus on content help to clarify issues, provide more information, and define problems. Interventions that focus on process aid in exploring or uncovering feelings and revealing themes or patterns of interaction. For example, if the therapist notices that family members are discussing a very emotionally charged issue with an absence of feeling, the therapist might intervene to identify this process. Solid therapeutic interventions involve both content and process.

A therapist considers several critical factors when choosing interventions. The timing of the intervention must be considered in evaluating its effectiveness. Timing affects how a particular strategy, a homework assignment, or a directive will be received by the family. Using a particular intervention too early in therapy, when there is insufficient trust in either the therapist or the process, can cause the intervention to fail.

In addition to trust, it is helpful to consider motivation for change in determining appropriate timing. If a client is highly motivated, he or she likely will be more receptive to interventions that accentuate change. If the client is resistant to change, then interventions that pace the client, such as tracking and active listening, might be in order. In the initial therapy session, where the primary goal is assessment, a "no change" stance can be beneficial. The "no change" stance assumes that until the therapist has completed an adequate assessment, introducing change is premature. It really does not make good therapeutic sense to suggest change before fully comprehending the problem.

Assessing and managing anxiety in a session can prove helpful in evaluating the choice of an intervention. Some interventions, such as open-ended questions, can increase a client's anxiety simply because the client doesn't immediately know the answer. Questions that are more orienting in nature, such as basic information regarding family or work history, are likely to decrease anxiety. A moderate level of anxiety is to be expected in therapy and assist in moving toward change. It is helpful for the therapist to note the level of anxiety in the session and anticipate which interventions are likely to heighten or diminish it.

Providing solid therapy and using interventions artfully take time and experience. Many factors comingle to determine the outcome. Good therapy is like good art—basics need to be mastered first: understanding yourself, your clients, and your context at multiple levels provides the setting in which a masterpiece is created.

Know Your Role in the Therapy

A number of essential responsibilities and aspects of the therapist's role are common to whatever theoretical approach is practiced. Some defining characteristics of the therapist's role have been spelled out legally, while others are part of the professional tradition. At the heart of it all is that the therapist has full responsibility for the therapy and the relationship.

It is the therapist's job to provide a structure, including a time, a place, and a format for clients to safely talk about their concerns. Basic responsibilities include being on time for therapy sessions, maintaining a professional posture in the relationship (including dress and demeanor), following through on information you promise to offer in therapy (such as psychoeducational resources or referrals), remembering to ask about homework assignments, and taking responsibility for structuring the therapeutic time together (ending on time, reviewing treatment goals as needed, stopping an escalating argument), all of which strengthen the working relationship.

The therapist is also responsible for determining the format of therapy, including rules for the communication process, such as each person having a turn to talk and be heard. In very chaotic or volatile cases, the therapist may need to closely monitor the communication to assist the family in developing more effective communication skills. He or she may choose to initiate discussion of how material from the sessions will be used outside therapy. Again, the therapeutic environment needs to include an umbrella of safety; it may be useful to suggest to clients that certain topics are best discussed in therapy, at least until the family develops more effective communication skills.

Beyond these practical matters, therapist responsibility has been clarified many times in legal principles like confidentiality, dual relationships, and duty to warn. The law holds the therapist completely responsible for establishing the boundaries of the relationship. He or she must spell out what clients can and cannot expect from therapy and from the therapist.

Another aspect of the therapist's role is to ensure that the relationship with the client is one-sided: the content of the therapy is about the client, therapeutic goals are about the client, and self-disclosure is generally done by the client. Instead of seeking mutuality in the relationship, the therapist cares for the client and focuses on his or her problems. However, therapists may choose to make certain self-disclosures in a therapeutic context.

Therapists' disclosure of personal information will vary according to each one's personal style and theoretical framework. Some theories, such as experiential therapy, will utilize more self-disclosure than others. Personal style in self-disclosure may be indicated by how intimately a therapist decorates the office (for example, with photographs of spouse and children) and how directly he or she answers a client's questions about his or her own family life.

A therapist should consider some of the following guidelines in determining level of self-disclosure:

1. The therapeutic relationship, like any relationship, takes some time to develop. It is more appropriate to talk more personally about yourself after you've known someone for a longer time.

2. Most therapists self-disclose more freely with children and adolescents. These clients tend to equate self-disclosure with a measure of trust. They will ask more personal questions than adults and appear to be curious about the therapist.

3. Therapist credibility may be enhanced by self-disclosure of information about one's educational or professional credentials.

4. A therapist should keep in mind that self-disclosure may impact each client differently. Some clients will be more comfortable with a professional distance wherein self-disclosure is kept to a minimum, and others will prefer to know something about the therapist before they feel comfortable opening up about themselves.

5. A therapist should only disclose personal information that has been thought about and processed, and avoid current issues that are creating personal turmoil.

The therapist must consider the impact of self-disclosure on the client. Providing information about oneself such as educational background or professional training can by very helpful in joining with a client and increasing confidence in the therapeutic process. Sometimes clients will ask personal questions, perhaps about marital status or whether or not you have children, and this can also be helpful in joining and in creating rapport. A therapist can offer personal reactions or feelings to a situation, such as being concerned about a client's well-being, as a leading statement to help generate a reaction from the client. A therapist may offer a story about his or her life or something that happened to someone else in order to stimulate the client's thinking or offer an alternative perspective on an issue. However, the therapist also may get caught in his or her own reactions to a client and share feelings inappropriately, which might indicate that the therapist has lost direction in the therapeutic process.

It's helpful for the therapist to understand his or her own intentions in self-disclosing personal information and reactions, and attempt to anticipate the impact on the client. A couple coming to marital therapy may not benefit from knowing that their therapist is currently in the process of divorcing. In another case, it may be helpful for the therapist to normalize a couple's difficulty in coping with new parenthood by discussing personal experiences. Clearly, the degree to which a therapist's role encompasses sharing is driven by a combination of personal preference, theoretical orientation, and client considerations.

Finally, it is part of the therapist's role to demonstrate some knowledge and expertise about the client's problem. Clients expect therapists to provide guidance and knowledge. This expectation is sometimes intimidating for beginning therapists. For example, if they are young, unmarried, and don't have children or lack some other quality or characteristic, the clients may question their expertise. The therapist must address this concern in a non-defensive manner. Such issues of credibility—and how beginning therapists can deal with it, are discussed in detail in Chapter 3. Beginning therapists should remember that they *do* have knowledge most clients don't have. Helping clients understand how cognitive-behavioral therapy helps depression or asking questions that reveal forgotten solutions are among the many ways beginning therapists demonstrate their knowledge.

Having discussed some commonalities, it's important to recognize significant variations in how therapists define their roles. These differences are influenced by the therapist's personality, the client's personality, the presenting problem, the client's emotional needs, and a variety of other factors. For one, the therapist's theoretical orientation can strongly influence how he or she views her role. An experiential family therapist is more likely than a behavioral family therapist to view some self-disclosure as acceptable. Narrative therapists are more likely to take a collaborative stance than are strategic family therapists.

The client's situation and needs also help define the therapist's role. A couple who come for therapy because the death of their child is destroying their marriage need a different kind of therapeutic relationship than a family whose presenting problem is their child's defiant behavior. In the first case, the therapist might define his or her role as being a source of intense emotional support during a time of sorrow, and acknowledge the strong attachment and dependence that the clients have on the therapy and therapist. In the second case, the therapist might act more like a consultant—staying in the periphery of the family interaction and only commenting periodically.

Therapists vary significantly in their beliefs about their role, which determine whether they accept gifts from clients, go to clients' weddings and funerals, and have pictures of their family in their office. Generally, therapists with a psychoanalytic background are more sensitive to transference issues and less likely to share any personal information either directly or indirectly. Beginning therapists can talk to their supervisors and teachers about these issues and will likely discover wide variation in response. For some of these issues, there is no clear answer. However, it is useful to understand the premises underlying the supervisor's opinion, which usually relate to how the supervisor views his or her own role as a therapist.

Although this discussion has been devoted to the therapist's role and responsibilities, remember that clients carry some responsibility as well—their behavior and for making their own decisions. The therapist's role is to guide clients, not to make decisions for them. If a client decides to enter into a relationship that may be personally destructive, that decision needs to be respected by the therapist. He or she may offer alternatives or look at the client's motivation in entering into the relationship, but, ultimately, it is the client's choice. The client has to live with it. Finally, clients are responsible for bringing their concerns to therapy and maintaining some respect for the process. The therapy will likely be more productive if the client comes prepared to talk about issues of current concern.

Create Family Therapy Treatment Plans

Family therapists need to develop a way to document what they do in relational terms, as it is this emphasis that characterizes family therapy. In Chapter 5, we reviewed the initial treatment plan and its usefulness in organizing your work. A key treatment skill for family therapists is the ability to write a thorough treatment plan. The one offered in this section contains some of the same steps as those discussed in the previous chapter, but differs in the specificity of behavioral or other measurable terms. As you recall, the seven treatment plan steps include (1) selecting a problem list; (2) examining history of the problems and previous/current treatment; (3) making a diagnosis using a DSM-IV multiaxial assessment; (4) establishing long-term goals; (5) choosing treatment modality, objectives, and interventions; (6) determining length and frequency of treatment; and (7) considering referral to outside resources.

Step 1 lists the problems using specific behavioral language, and thus, measurable terms. For example, rather than stating a problem such as "anxiety," you might write "frequent feelings of panic, fear, and helplessness when faced with being alone." Step 2 notes the history of the problems and previous or current treatment resources, as in the initial treatment plan. Step 3 provides a five-axis diagnosis using DSM-IV categories. The multiaxial assessment includes clinical disorders, personality disorders, general medical conditions, psychosocial and environmental problems, and global assessment of functioning. Step 4 offers several global, long-term goals needed to address the problem. The goals indicate the desired, positive outcome of treatment. Step 5 specifies the modality of treatment—either individual, couple, family, or group—and measurable treatment objectives for each goal and associated interventions. In contrast to long-term goals, objectives must be stated in behaviorally measurable words. At least two objectives need to be written for each longer-term goal. The words "increase" or "decrease," when associated with specific behaviors such as arguing or communicating, will fit well here. Interventions tied to each objective come next. For example, the clinician may ask a family member to keep track of each argument the family has and bring the list to therapy. If an intervention is not successful, others may be added to the treatment plan. As discussed in Chapter 5, interventions stem from a selected family therapy theoretical perspective. Step 6 notes the length and frequency of treatment. An estimate of the number of sessions needed is given. Step 7 considers referrals to outside community and professional resources. Table 6.1 shows what a final plan might look like after the preceding issues have been addressed.

TABLE 6.1. Sample Family Therapy Treatment Plan

Step 1: Select a problem list.

1. Use of verbally abusive language when talking to others, especially partner.
2. History of throwing household objects and breaking things during arguments.
3. History of hostile outbursts in social situations.
4. Frequent arguing with spouse.

Step 2: Examine history of problems and previous/current treatment.

Client history of hostility since adolescence, most often while intoxicated. No previous history of therapy. Client actively participating in Alcoholics Anonymous for 2 years.

Step 3: Make a diagnosis (DSM-IV).

Axis I: 312.34 Intermittent Explosive Disorder
          305.0 Alcohol Abuse in Full Remission
Axis II: None
Axis III: High Blood Pressure
Axis IV: Moderate Psychosocial Stressors
Axis V: 60 (moderate difficulty in social functioning)

Step 4: Establish long-term goals.

1. Increase awareness of client's and partner's role in relationship conflicts.
2. Develop the ability to handle conflicts in a mature, controlled, nonaggressive and/or assertive way.
3. Develop skills for effective and mutually satisfying communication within the relationship.

Step 5: Choose treatment modality, objectives, and interventions.

Conjoint therapy using primarily strategic and behavioral interventions.

Objectives	Interventions
1a. Increase awareness of anger expression patterns.	Assign clients book, *Intimate Enemy* (Finley, 1997).
1b. Identify escalating interactional cycles.	Review common fight sequences. Visually display pattern.
2a. Decrease the intensity and frequency of conflictual interactions within relationship.	Assign clients to talk daily about prechosen, nonemotional topics for 5 minutes without arguing; increase time and degree of depth with success; assign time to fight with each other.
2b. Identify and verbalize needs both partners have in relationship.	Train and practice communication skills; list and verbalize needs.
3a. Discuss the level of intimacy; increase time in enjoyable contact.	Assign clients to identify positive interactional sequences; assign shared social activities.

Step 6: Determine length and frequency of treatment.

Weekly couple therapy for eight sessions; bimonthly sessions for six more meetings; total of 14 sessions to be completed in 6 months.

Step 7: Consider referral to outside resources.

Continued attendance in Alcoholics Anonymous.

Recent resources such as the book *The Complete Psychotherapy Treatment Planner* (Jongsma & Peterson, 1996) or the computerized treatment planning program *TheraScribe for Windows* can help you organize and develop treatment plans that individually match your clients' needs. The family therapist balances the relational, therapeutic, and ethical concerns of practice. It is a taxing role, yet very rewarding. Creativity and professional knowledge combine to help persons in the healing process. The basic treatment skills discussed must be coordinated with the art of matching these skills to particular clients with particular problems, keeping in mind the kind of therapist you are. This is a lifelong and challenging component of being a family therapist. We close this chapter on treatment skills by offering, in Table 6.2, a list of self-assessment questions. Beginning therapists may find these helpful in gauging and guiding their early work.

TABLE 6.2. Self-Assessment Questions Regarding Treatment Skills

To create a therapeutic relationship

1. Do I show a concerned interest for my clients?
2. Have I structured a safe therapeutic environment in the room and set guidelines for working outside of the session?
3. Can I understand my clients' experience to some extent at both emotional and cognitive levels?
4. Do I continue to be curious about this case?
5. Do I need to be clear about my status as a trainee or intern, or my lack of expertise in a particular area?

To assess and intervene

1. Do I ask the appropriate questions to assess (e.g., lineal and circular questions) and intervene (e.g., strategic and reflexive questions)?
2. Can I normalize the clients' concerns in some way?
3. Will reframing the presenting problem help to change the way it is understood?
4. Do the clients perceive me as increasing their social support system?
5. Can I confront the family when necessary?
6. Am I aware of the pacing needs for these clients?
7. Have I considered referrals that would be useful?
8. Would psychoeducational material (e.g. reading, handouts, Internet website) be useful for these clients?
9. Do I have a treatment plan in place?

To develop my family therapy skills

1. Am I clear about my theoretical approach?
2. Do my interventions match my theoretical understanding of the problem?
3. Would it be useful to read an article or chapter on this treatment approach or problem? Do I need to attend a workshop soon?
4. Have I consulted with a colleague or supervisor if I get confused?
5. Am I managing the legal and ethical concerns of this case well?

7

Working with Families
and Children

Lisa S sat wide-eyed and trembling on the edge of her chair, occasionally hiding with one hand a persistent tic in her left eye. It was her first visit to a therapist's office, and since 9-year-old Lisa was by nature a shy and nervous child, she left the talking to her mother and father. Mr. and Mrs. S leaned toward the therapist, and painfully revealed their daughter's daily panic attacks and their own frustration in trying to solve Lisa's "problem." By the end of the interview, the therapist had compiled a rich history and a number of hypotheses about Lisa's disorder. Although Lisa was clearly the identified patient (IP), there was no question that family work would be part of treatment. Having carefully listened to and empathized with his new clients, the therapist began to talk teamwork. . . .

Perhaps our deepest conviction in working with children is that, with remarkably few exceptions, primary caretakers are absolutely key to the assessment and effective treatment of childhood disorders. This "umbrella" assumption might appear obvious to those who define themselves as "family therapists," but in fact it covers a significantly broader field and, in so doing, helps keep us oriented to some crucial facts:

1. Without caretakers as cotherapists, our interventions with children may become 50-minute exercises whose impact quickly dissipates in the 10,000 minutes that lie between sessions.
2. Whether we lean toward a view of childhood problems as somehow functional within the family or are inclined to see childhood

118

disorders from a more individual perspective, our work with children almost always involves addressing the hopes, fears, attitudes, and abilities of the grownups with whom our child clients live. Indeed, a collaborative set in which parents or primary caretakers share their own "assessments" and carry insights, information, and actions "learned" in therapy into the home is basic.

With this single principle to guide us, we present in this chapter a brief discussion of assessment issues with children, recent research findings regarding family interventions, and some pointers for working with children and their families at various life cycle and developmental stages. Finally, we complete the chapter with comments regarding special considerations for divorcing and remarried families, mediation and child custody evaluation, and the challenges of helping disadvantaged single-parent families.

ASSESSMENT OF CHILD AND ADOLESCENT DISORDERS

Art historians are likely familiar with that period of time in which European painters depicted children as miniature adults. Similarly, sociologists and anthropologists report on those eras in which children were surmised to think, feel, and behave as adults in undersized bodies. Today, of course, the differentiation between "child" and "adult" is as complex as it is well documented. In psychopathology, however, we continue a struggle to define, identify, and treat mental disorders that, previously described and treated among adults, behave quite differently in children.

In our work on an inpatient psychiatric facility for children, we are reminded daily of how childhood itself complicates differential diagnoses. The common behavioral symptoms seen in troubled children cut across neat diagnostic categories and, in so doing, engage all our skills of assessment and appropriate treatment planning: "Are this child's mood swings a sign of ADHD? Bipolar disorder? Should a DSM-IV diagnosis even be made? Or are these symptoms an offshoot of marital conflict and 'poor' parenting?" In any case, diagnoses are made with caution, and assessment is ongoing and comprehensive, involving the biological (e.g., electroencephalograms [EEGs] and magnetic resonance imaging [MRIs] to detect brain abnormalities), the social (detailed information gathering regarding family, school, and peer relationships), and the psychological (use of paper-and-pencil instruments and projective tests).

While a biopsychosocial approach enriches our assessment of childhood *and* adult disorders, we cannot underestimate the importance of assessing family issues, particularly when the IP is a youngster. Estrada and Pinsof (1995) point out the growing influence of a systems view in child assessment by noting the following common premises: (1) the view of child and family disorders as constellations of interrelated systems and subsystems; (2) the need to consider the entire family situation when assessing the impact of any single variable; (3) the idea that similar behavior may be the result of different sets of initiating factors; (4) a recognition that intervention is likely to lead to multiple outcomes, including readjustment of relationships within the family system; and (5) the notion that family systems and subsystems possess dynamic properties and are constantly changing over time (p. 405).

In addition, a growing body of literature suggests that the development of child and adolescent problems does not occur in a vacuum but is strongly influenced by certain marital and family characteristics. For example, factors such as marital discord, parental psychopathology, social-cognitive deficits in family members, socioeconomic disadvantage, disrupted parent–child relations, lack of social support, and social isolation are all variables that strongly influence the course of a child's individual disorder. This literature gives a strong argument for a systemic assessment.

Having considered these important family variables, the therapist working with Lisa S and her parents would have discovered some enlightening facts and expanded his hypotheses for later treatment. We learn, for example, that Lisa's father has a history of panic attack and agoraphobia; that both parents are inadvertently maintaining Lisa's symptoms by avoiding using the words "death" or "dying," which often precipitate attacks; that Mr. S has unresolved grief issues from a death in his family; that Mr. and Mrs. S disagree strongly about how to parent their daughter, but avoid discussions or arguments about these differences. We also find that about the time Lisa's attacks began, her father had lost his job due to his agoraphobia and a role change had occurred in which Dad now stayed home to care for Lisa and Mom left the house to work.

Certainly, individual assessment and diagnosis of children is important. In Lisa's case, we can utilize DSM-IV and find that our client meets the criteria for panic attack. Based purely on individual symptoms reported by Lisa and her parents, we can then design a treatment program based on known effective interventions for anxiety disorders. However, by taking a systemic as well as an individual approach in our evaluation, we can supplement Lisa's treatment by addressing the family issues that clearly impact her symptoms. Thus, our assessment has expanded and enriched the treatment.

While family therapists are primarily concerned with systemic assessment and intervention, it will be increasingly important for all clinicians to have an up-to-date and working knowledge of individual diagnoses for children and adolescents. For example, a familiarity with such common childhood diagnoses as depression, behavioral or attention-deficit/hyper-activity disorders, pervasive developmental disorders (autism), and con-duct disorders is expected. Other problems that are frequently diagnosed in children and adolescents include fear and anxiety disorders (especially phobias), and substance abuse. Many children have problems that are comorbid. For example, a young child may be diagnosed with attention-deficit/hyperactivity disorder, and later be diagnosed with a conduct dis-order and substance abuse problem.

It is beyond the scope of this section to describe in detail the diagnos-tic criteria for each child and adolescent disorder. A brief summary is presented in Table 7.1.

Family therapists are well advised to become familiar with such in-struments as the Child Behavior Checklist (See Connors, 1987), in which multiple sources provide information about a child's behavior, and the Connors, a neuropsychosocial instrument for assessing hyperactive chil-dren (Connors, 1987). In addition, since child and adolescent assessment often focuses on development, many pencil-and-paper instruments and projective "tests" are used to assess intelligence and development: the Wechsler Intelligence Scale for Children, third edition (WISC-III; Wechsler, 1991), the draw-a-person test, and the house–tree–person tests (Buck & Jolles, 1966). Many of these tests are used in the educational batteries of school districts. While most family therapists will not be administering these instruments as part of their therapy, it is important that they know about what psychological evaluation instruments are available and make appropriate referrals for further evaluation, especially when they suspect a child has a developmental disorder or other learning problem.

FAMILY INTERVENTIONS WHEN CHILDREN ARE THE CLIENTS

Beginning therapists often struggle with how to do family therapy when the client is 4 years old and isn't inclined to disclose concerns or talk about feelings. While various forms of play therapy and other projective ap-proaches help a child express or work through problems, we return to our guiding principle—effective therapy, especially with children, will rely on helping parents or caretakers become engaged in the process, clarify their own roles in the family, and become cotherapists who conduct their own interventions at home.

In choosing specific treatment approaches for families with children, beginning therapists can be guided by what we know so far. In this sec-tion, we provide a brief glimpse of family treatments that have been stud-ied and supported by research. Later, we highlight key developmental

TABLE 7.1. Common Childhood Disorders

Category of disorder	Essential features
Attention-deficit/ hyperactivity disorder	1. Inattention: inability to finish activities that require concentration at school, home, or play; doesn't seem to listen; easily distracted. 2. Hyperactivity: excessive activity; fidgets excessively; can't sit still. 3. Impulsivity: impatience; difficulty waiting for one's turn; interrupts or intrudes excessively. 4. Behavioral manifestations occur in more than one setting, were present before age 7, and impair developmentally appropriate functioning.
Conduct disorder	1. Violation of basic rights of others, norms, or rules. 2. Behaviors includes some or all of the following: aggression toward people and animals; destruction of property; deceitfulness or theft; and serious violation of rules (truancy, running away).
Pervasive developmental disorder (autism)	1. Impaired social interaction: doesn't respond to others nonverbally (i.e., eye contact is lacking); doesn't seek interaction. 2. Impaired communication: delay in, or lack of, speech; stereotyped use of language; idiosyncratic use of language. 3. Restricted, repetitive behaviors: abnormally intense preoccupation with object or activity; inflexible adherence to rituals or routine; repetitive motor movements.
Attachment disorders (separation anxiety and reactive attachment disorders)	1. In separation anxiety: excessive anxiety about being away from home or from person to whom child is attached; distress or worry about losing other; fear and/or reluctance about sleeping alone, going to school; nightmares. 2. In reactive attachment disorder: failure to thrive; pathogenic care (neglect); excessive inhibition, hypervigilance, or ambivalence in social interactions.
Depression	1. Depressed or irritable mood: feelings of sadness, hopelessness, worthlessness, guilt. 2. Loss of interest in activities once enjoyed. 3. Loss of energy: fatigue, inability to concentrate. 4. Change in appetite: failure to make expected weight gains. 5. Change in sleep: insomnia or hypersomnia. 6. Recurrent thoughts of death: suicidal ideation.

issues throughout the family life cycle and how these inform treatment decisions.

Much of the child and adolescent treatment literature draws on the parent management training (PMT) model developed by Gerald Patterson at the University of Oregon. This model was originally developed for work with antisocial youth but has now been applied to a range of childhood disorders. The underlying assumption of the model is that behavior problems are inadvertently developed and maintained by maladaptive parent–child interactions. Therapists teach parents to use specific skills when interacting with their children, in order to promote prosocial behavior and to decrease deviant behavior (Estrada & Pinsof, 1995).

Among the common characteristics shared by all PMT treatments are the following: (1) The treatment is conducted by parents who directly implement procedures in the home; (2) parents learn to identify, define, and observe problem behavior; (3) the treatment sessions cover social learning principles including positive reinforcement, punishment, negotiation, and contingency contracting; (4) these strategies are taught through a prescribed set of therapy activities including modeling and role playing; and (5) the program's goal is development of specific parenting skills.

Estrada and Pinsof (1995) report that PMT is probably the most widely used family intervention in the treatment of childhood disorders. Their review of 20 years' worth of empirical research demonstrates these and other findings in the study of common disorders of children:

1. *Conduct disorders* (including oppositional defiant disorder): Family therapy, especially PMT, is an effective treatment for families and children with conduct disorders. Maintenance of these improvements is still an issue; continuation of the gains made appears to be moderated by other factors, such as marital distress, social isolation, or other variables.

2. *Attention-deficit/hyperactivity disorder* (ADHD): Family interventions, particularly PMT, improve child management skills. Parents report increased confidence, reduced stress, and improved family relationships. Research demonstrates a reduction in children's noncompliance and aggression rather than in core symptoms such as inattention, impulsivity, and overactivity. Research definitely supports the use of medication to treat ADHD. Longer-term, combined behavioral–medication treatments have the most lasting effects.

3. *Fears and anxiety disorders*: Anxiety problems are the most common psychological problems reported by children, and many adults with anxiety disorders report their problems started in childhood. These disorders include school phobias and other phobias such as fear of the dark, of medical visits, and of separation from parents. Research yields tentative

support for the efficacy of approaches that involve parents in the treatment of their children's fear and anxiety.

4. *Pervasive developmental disorders* (autistic disorder): Autistic disorder is the only developmental disorder with a clear body of family research supporting its efficacy. Autism research focuses on training a child's parents to serve as teachers and therapists, and it suggests that families with autistic children can achieve lasting gains from family-based interventions. Families that fare the best have the least cognitively impaired children (mental retardation is common in children with autism). They also have families that can participate in a demanding treatment program, as well as support from schools that encourage parent training efforts at home.

Along with empirical findings, such as the research pointing to the efficacy of involving the family in interventions for childhood disorders (Estrada & Pinsof, 1995), family therapy clinicians are guided by theoretical concepts, such as the formulations of the family life cycle, that help inform their assessment and treatment of client families. Clearly, information on developmental issues is not enough to conduct effective family therapy, but understanding what we can expect of families and children at various stages and which issues are pressing for them from year to year is absolutely vital to our work.

THE FAMILY LIFE CYCLE REVISITED

Early studies of the family (Duvall, 1955) clearly noted that the ages of its members impacted the differing tasks of the family. Synthesizing these observations and applying this information to the needs of the family therapist, Carter and McGoldrick (1989) categorized the family life cycle into six stages with a key emotional process and several developmental examples at each stage (see Table 7.2).

The systemic backdrop to these ideas stems from the assumption that the family must go through a second-order change at each developmental stage for its members to proceed in a healthy way. Second-order change necessitates a redefining of the family system at behavioral, cognitive, emotional, and relational domains. A shift must occur over time.

Families often present to a therapist when they are in the midst of these developmental shifts. The family therapist hypothesizes that the presenting problem may have a lot to do with the family being stuck in its progress toward achieving a particular developmental stage. For example, a 14-year-old daughter of very controlling parents may start "acting out" by breaking curfew and hanging out at school with people the parents

TABLE 7.2. The Stages of the Family Life Cycle

Family life cycle stage	Emotional process of transition: Key principles	Second-order changes in family status required to proceed developmentally
1. Leaving home: Single, young adults	Accepting emotional and financial responsibility for self	a. Differentiation of self in relation to family of origin b. Development of intimate peer relationships c. Establishment of self re work and financial independence
2. The joining of families through marriage: The new couple	Commitment to new system	a. Formulation of marital system b. Realignment of relationships with extended families and friends to include spouse
3. Families with young children	Accepting new members into the system	a. Adjusting marital system to make space for child(ren) b. Joining in childrearing, financial, and household tasks c. Realignment of relationships with extended family to include parenting and grandparenting roles
4. Families with adolescents	Increasing flexibility of family boundaries to include children's independence and grandparents' frailties	a. Shifting of parent–child relationships to permit adolescent to move in and out of system b. Refocus on midlife marital and career issues c. Beginning shift toward joint caring for older generation
5. Launching children and moving on	Accepting a multitude of exits from and entries into the family system	a. Renegotiation of marital system as a dyad b. Development of adult to adult relationships between grown children and their parents c. Realignment of relationships to include in-laws and grandchildren d. Dealing with disabilities and death of parents (grandparents)
6. Families in later life	Accepting the shifting of generational roles	a. Maintaining own and/or couple functioning and interests in face of psychological decline; exploration of new familial and social role options b. Support for a more central role of middle generation c. Making room in the system for the wisdom and experience of the elderly, supporting the older generation without overfunctioning for them d. Dealing with loss of spouse, siblings, and other peers and preparation for own death. Life review and integration.

Note. From B. Carter and M. McGoldrick, *The Changing Family Life Cycle.* Copyright 1989 by Allyn & Bacon. Reprinted by permission.

deem unacceptable. This behavior signals a difficulty in the family system's shift to the "family with adolescents" stage, where there is a need to increase the flexibility of the family boundary to include the teenager's growing independence.

The first task at each transitional stage is for the therapist to normalize what is going on in the family, framing many of the presenting problems as common and understandable. A therapist can use the life cycle information to connect more fully with the family, as it helps him to understand their dilemmas more completely. In normalizing, a therapist must be careful not to trivialize the pain, fears, and emotional power of these developmental shifts. When done well, normalizing can be offered as a first "gift" to the family from the therapist, toning down the emotional turmoil within the family. The therapist's expertise in understanding what the family is about helps establish a solid working alliance. Thus, life cycle information boosts the therapist's authority, which is especially helpful if he's significantly younger than the other adults in the therapy room.

Knowing the key emotional task at each developmental stage provides guidance to the therapist. What must the family members affectively manage in order to proceed? Therapists can connect to family members' deeper emotional issues by using information in the family life cycle. For example, the key emotional transition for two individuals to make in forming a marriage is "commitment to a new system." Without a new system that cultivates a place for each partner to be included and respected, a kind of competition takes place wherein each person attempts to win the battle for dominion over a particular area of life, be it housecleaning, finances, or friendships. A therapist, aware of the necessary emotional transition, can direct the couple to find ways in which each person can be comfortable with a decision. The therapist facilitates the couple's transition from a "me" to a "we."

Second-order changes may be noted at each developmental juncture. For example, at the couple stage core tasks include formation of the couple system and reorganization of relationships with friends and relatives. Specific tasks often need to be accomplished before a given stage has been mastered. Here we must caution the therapist to culturally determine the behaviors at each stage. A Hispanic couple may stay more physically and emotionally connected to their families than a middle-class Anglo couple would throughout the lifespan. Both have formed a couple system, but the style of reorganization with relatives might differ significantly.

The following sections highlight core areas to remember at each developmental stage and some practical ways the therapist can manage family members. Each section refers to basic family life cycle concerns.

Young Children, Birth to 4 Years

Frank and Laura were on the verge of divorce when they agreed, as a last resort, to give therapy a try. With their 19-month-old daughter in tow, it soon became apparent to the therapist that the couple's smooth sailing days had ended when they struck the rocky shores of new parenthood. Since the birth of their baby and Laura's 6-week maternity leave, the couple continued their prebaby work schedule. The baby was put into quality home childcare, but Mom and Dad felt guilty about this and spent all of their evening hours and weekend time devoted to their little girl. Before long, chronic crankiness (of the parents, not the baby!) deteriorated into outright fighting. Frank and Laura had a hard time remembering why they married in the first place. Clearly, without a renegotiation of their adult, "couple space," divorce looked imminent.

This couple's story is a reminder that marital issues are paramount in this stage of the family life cycle. New parents must take time and energy to develop an emotional attachment to the baby, as well as meet his or her physical needs. A family's response to the new baby can range from a "hardly noticing" to a "drop everything" stance. In the former, or closed boundary stance, the parent or couple won't be able to meet the needs of a very dependent child since a baby requires significant family resources. Neglect of one form or another can result. On the "drop everything" end of the spectrum, a family opens its arms wide to the child at the expense of all other relationships, including the couple's own. Though well suited for the very early aspects of this stage, a child-centered family often struggles with the growing independence needs of its members at later stages of the family life cycle. Problems of marital distress or individual functioning (depression) could result.

Fights over child rearing, household tasks, and financial responsibilities are common at this stage. Particularly when couples haven't formed a new system in the previous stage of the family life cycle (the joining of families), the practical urgency and plentitude of stressors and decisions here can seem overwhelming. Gender issues often come to the forefront at this stage, too. Sue and Joe, who lived together for 5 years, had been separated for 2 weeks when they sought therapy. Their 4-year-old son and 2-year-old daughter were the motivation behind this move, yet as we explored what brought them in, the couple's children seemed to comprise the major battleground. Both Sue and Joe needed to work in order to make their rent payments, but Sue resented this, saying that Joe doesn't make as much money as he could in his sales work. Sue, whose mother stayed home until Sue was in sixth grade, longed to be able to do the same. Joe, raised by his Mom in a single-parent household, believed Sue needed to work in order to provide their children with a house and yard he never had. Clashes about role expectations, especially gender role expectations, come to a powerful crescendo at this stage.

An understanding of these practical, emotional, and interpersonal issues that appear in families with very young children can guide therapeutic interventions and help new parents make a successful transition from one life cycle stage to the next.

While this early phase of family life brings more parents to therapy than children, therapists will occasionally meet with families whose IP is an infant or toddler. Three-year-old Jason came to therapy for repeated aggressive behavior against his 1-year-old sibling, for destroying toys and for household belongings, and trying to climb out of a moving car. His single mother presented Jason to the therapist with a simple plea: "I don't know why he does it! But you've got to make it stop!" Clearly, how the therapist explores Jason's problems and ultimately how he or she treats them are limited by Jason's age.

Family therapists who work with very young children can base their initial assessment and treatment on the child's developmental stage. The literature on children's emotional, cognitive, and social development from infancy to adulthood is voluminous, and we would do a disservice to its scholars to encapsulate developmental theory here. While we encourage beginning therapists to learn about or refresh themselves on the needs and expectations of each stage of childhood and adolescence, our focus is on brief reminders about developmental issues and practical steps to take when a young child toddles into your office.

Armed with the knowledge that infants and toddlers require secure attachments in order to build a trustful orientation toward life, we can assess very young children in terms of their early attachments and the sense of autonomy they show, among other variables. Our knowledge about cognitive development also shapes our expectations: for example, realizing that "time out" can be understood by a toddler, while "telling the truth" is much less clear to someone who is 3 years old. In Jason's case, for example, we learned that frequent separations from his mother and maltreatment by intermittent caretakers marked this youngster's first years of life. Further, his mother's ignorance of the cognitive capabilities of her toddler likely made the situation at home more difficult. Lengthy "explanations" of why siblings should not be hit or thrown had little impact on Jason's aggressive behavior. Immediately, we have clues to the route family therapy can take—reestablishing a secure attachment between Jason and his mother, and helping this single parent learn appropriate methods of dealing with her child's behavior.

Beginning therapists can also benefit from a number of practical guidelines for working with very young children. These involve space, safety, shared responsibility, and expectations.

Space

Most therapy offices don't fit the needs of both adults and children. Traditional play therapy rooms may be too cramped or full of potential hazards (paint, clay) for an adult to relax. In contrast, immovable, adult-oriented rooms may paralyze and increase anxiety in children. Ideally, therapy rooms should accommodate full family interactions as well as provide separate spaces for play and for separating out family subsystems, if needed. A larger room, sparsely furnished with movable chairs and pillows could accommodate all. It's also helpful to have play areas with toys that encourage interaction between children and adults (hand puppets, crayons and paper, simple games). All of these assist therapy.

Safety

Safety needs to be established during the therapy session, and everybody can help make this possible. Therapists need to check the therapy room and remove or "childproof" potentially dangerous items before the session starts. Parents often believe the therapist will take responsibility for setting limits and discipline during the session. It's helpful to assign the major responsibilities to the parents instead, using rules they have at home. This offers a way to strengthen the parental position in the family hierarchy and gives the therapist an opportunity to see how the family functions.

Shared Responsibility

Although setting a collaborative tone with most families is helpful, allowing for a flexible sharing of the work with young children is essential. Therapists need to be able to sit on the floor and play with the children when this activity is useful. Parents can take their child for a walk as a break when necessary. Often cotherapy teams can assist greatly in managing the subsystems of a particular family. One therapist can take a child into another room, while the other therapist works with the parent. Also, selecting session times that don't interfere with naps and mealtimes is helpful. Asking parents to bring a favorite toy might be useful, too. Finally, creatively dividing up the family system for different sessions over time—one oriented for a parent–child focus, one for parents only—can assist in better management of therapeutic goals.

Expectations

For children in particular, nothing is sacred about weekly, 50-minute therapy sessions. Shorter or longer sessions or meetings divided into smaller segments can help the therapist's work with a family. Toddlers, in particular, will rarely be able to sit for more than a few minutes of talk necessitating the need for play therapy involving games, artwork, or storytelling. Action in the therapy session and participation between family members is also helpful for older children and adults. In addition, family therapy often makes sense as "brief therapy." After a longer intake/assessment session, for example, a therapist might offer several interventions to be tried out over several weeks and request the family report the results at a later session. Home visits, too, can often result in very helpful information on ways of adapting the environment to alleviate problems with a young child. In short, flexibility and teamwork are crucial to working with families with very young children.

Children Ages 5–12 Years

Family life cycle concerns at this stage are similar to the previous ones in that they reflect a need to adapt to change. What often differs at this stage is the expansion of the family's contact with larger social systems. If children have been in half-day preschool, the transition now is to full-day school. If children have been in full-day child care, they now have full-day school and participation in sports activities after school and on weekends. Further, evaluation of the child now involves comparisons with peers, and the ability or inability of a child to "fit in" becomes more prominent. The school system connects intimately with the life of the family. Problems or successes at school can impact the family system.

During this and the previous stage, renegotiating relationship issues with extended family also takes place. What will be the role of the grandparents, aunts, uncles, and cousins? Previous issues within the family that haven't been resolved are revived during this time. For example, when molestation or other kinds of abuse have occurred in the family, fears and boundary concerns come to the fore. For parents, the issue in therapy may relate to contacts their children will have with relatives. Glenda presented to her therapist the dilemma of what to do when her mother invited her 8-year-old daughter to spend the night for a weekend. Glenda had been molested by her stepfather, who was still married to her mother. She had an ongoing relationship with her family, but always watched her daughter when grandfather was around. Glenda had worked on her past in group therapy but hadn't brought up her concerns to her family directly. Family therapists will frequently be called upon to help clients navigate through transgenerational difficulties at this stage.

For the children in this stage, the focus is around starting school, moving out into the world, and building self-esteem by managing their environment more intentionally. Feelings of being a failure or success permeate activities such as tying shoelaces and learning to read. Development of initiative versus guilt and industry versus inferiority provide the basis of many daily concerns for the child. Peer relationships become more and more central, and comparisons to others—"Tommy's the best kickball player at school" or "June can read two books a day"—seem to pervade many social interactions. The task for parents, teachers, and therapist is to find places where a child can experience competency and some level of proficiency. If this is not the case at school, parents can look to sports, art, music, and relationships outside school for experiences that will help a child develop a healthy self-concept.

It's not surprising to find therapy clinics brimming with 5-, 6-, and 7-year-old children whose first months at school have been met with frustration or failure. This is the time when problems with attention, hyperactivity, anxiety, oppositionalism, and learning become evident to those outside the family. Frequently, young children make their way into therapy on the recommendations of school teachers and counselors. In some cases, the mere suggestion by school authorities is all the impetus distraught parents need to finally seek help.

This is an important point for beginning therapists to remember. By the time parents bring their youngsters to therapy, they are well acquainted with their child's behavioral problems and have likely tried "every trick in the book" to solve them. It's not unusual for us to see parents who report being fed up, exhausted, angry, lost, guilty, and in myriad other states when they arrive in our offices. Frequently, these beleaguered parents want you— the therapist—to fix the problem. Returning to our guiding principle, however, we're reminded that without the parent as cotherapist, our chances of success are minimal. Our first task, then, is to support and join with the parents, to empathize with their struggle, and to enlist their expertise as we present the real need for a team approach. Whether the treatment plan focuses on parent management training (as is typical with problems involving very young children) or is combined with re-creating parent–child bonds and nurturing the warm relationships that often get lost in stressful circumstances, our ability to engage and work with parents is at the heart of therapy with these children.

At the same time, our sense is that therapy will progress further, and parents will commit more to the process, if we can creatively engage children at these ages—they are therapeutic allies, information resources, and affective conduits for the family. Probably the easiest way to involve children at this age is through drawing and role playing. Therapists who aren't able to create a child-centered therapy room can often hide a large art pad and markers for artistic purposes under the couch. A basket full of puppets, dolls, and dress-up items can facilitate interaction at multiple levels within the family.

As with younger children, action needs to replace talk during some of the therapeutic encounters. Sessions can be broken up into sections where the child is "excused" from the therapy (although still in the room) while the therapist talks with parents directly. Therapists must be sure to edit any information that would be inappropriate for the children to overhear. Children can then be reengaged toward the end of the session for a summary of what the family might do during the week to continue improvement. After a session, stickers or other small items to reward the child's participation might encourage involvement in the future.

Besides working with the family itself, therapists must be mindful of what other "system players" need to be involved for therapy to proceed effectively. For example, since at this stage therapy is often initiated due to school concerns, contact with a teacher or other school personnel can significantly enhance work in the family therapy session. Minuchin, Montalvo, Guerney, Rosman, and Schumer (1967) recognize that demands from multiple systems (family, child, and school) often create problems, rather than that the child is the problem.

Active information gathering from the school, childcare, or sports or religious organizations with which the family is involved can be useful in shaping appropriate interventions. Whether or not the presenting problem only occurs in one setting or across multiple settings helps the therapist to orient his or her approach with the family. The following case demonstrates how interventions involving outside settings are both important and beneficial.

Brittany was a 12-year-old girl enrolled in the seventh grade. She was brought to therapy by her parents because she was having problems in school. She had done well in elementary school, achieving mostly As and Bs. After entering junior high school she hadn't performed well academically, getting Cs and Ds at the end of the first semester. She complained that she didn't like most of her teachers. She would do most of her homework but often "forgot" to turn it in. The parents reported no problems at home. She did most of her chores when she was asked and enjoyed playing softball and playing piano.

Brittany was a soft-spoken, bright, and articulate girl who felt "badly" about her school performance. She blamed most of the problem on a couple of her teachers who, she said, "don't like me and are boring." She often felt intimidated by the teachers and the school environment. She found going to different classes and having lots of teachers to be disruptive and chaotic. She was also struggling with making new friends and was feeling that she didn't fit in. Her response to feeling overwhelmed by the new school environment was to withdraw. She became afraid of failing, so decided not to turn in her homework. The more she got behind in her classes the more her feelings of failure and futility increased.

The parents responded that they were "concerned, frustrated, and helpless" about Brittany's school problems. The father was often out of town because of his work and he didn't have enough contact with Brittany to "truly understand the problems." The mother was frustrated in her attempts to help Brittany. She had tried to help the girl with her homework, but they would end up quarreling. She felt that Brittany wasn't interested in talking about school and would either withdraw or become defensive. Brittany's mother had contacted the school counselor but felt that the counselor was of little help. The counselor suggested that Brittany might need a tutor and that her test scores indicated that Brittany was "full of potential and easily capable of doing the work."

The therapist began working with the family, although the father's attendance was sporadic due to his work commitments. Brittany and her mother had a fairly close relationship. They spent a fair amount of time together and genuinely enjoyed each other's company. They shared interests in music and sports, and played tennis together. Their primary difficulty revolved around Brittany's school problems and an inability to communicate without arguing about school.

Brittany was having considerable difficulty in making the adjustment from the stable elementary school environment to the fluctuating schedule at the junior high school. She felt insecure and overwhelmed by the constant changes in her classes, the lack of individual attention, and the sheer number of students. The therapist contacted the school counselor in an effort to increase the school's interest in Brittany, and to obtain more structure and stability for her. The counselor said the school would cooperate in providing weekly progress reports on Brittany's work. The counselor also agreed to provide a student mentor for Brittany. The mentor would be an eighth grader who could help tutor Brittany and help familiarize her with the school. The mother was encouraged to contact several of Brittany's teachers and coordinate their efforts in determining whether or not Brittany turned in her homework.

Brittany responded very positively to the structure and interest she was given. Her adjustment to the new school was slower than most students and she needed some special attention. The therapist was able to intervene to work as a liaison between the school and the family and to effect positive solutions to Brittany's adjustment.

Adolescents

The primary emotional task for families at this stage is increasing the family's boundary flexibility to allow for children's growing independence. Flexibility may or may not be characteristic of the family throughout its history. Often this stage also signals a time in which the growing frailties of grandparents must be considered.

Second only to the life cycle period with young children, this stage is associated with a high number of divorces. One reason is the convergence of many powerful and sometimes competing needs of family members. First, the adolescent must be permitted to move in and out of the family system more fluidly. Friendships and relationships outside take on growing significance and the family sometimes becomes secondary in the young person's life. When family values conflict with the teenager's behavioral choices, the family might over- or underrespond. In either case, family therapy can enhance positive adaptation to this stage.

Issues besides adolescence are present at this stage—midlife concerns for parents often come to the fore. Regrets, missed opportunities, possibilities for beginning new dreams, reassessing the quality of the marital relationship all add to the challenging "mix." Further, stresses from taking care of older parents emerge. Such caretaking consumes time and financial resources. Adults in these families often term themselves "caught in the middle" between the financial and emotional needs of their older and younger members. The following case illustrates the interplay between difficulties around adolescence and midlife issues:

The C family was having difficulty with their youngest child, 15-year-old Derrick, who hadn't been coming home at night, was doing poorly at school, and had been caught with marijuana on several occasions. Derrick was a star football player on his high school team. He was a bright, likeable, and outgoing young man who appeared self-assured. He came from a family of four children, in which the other three were out of the home—two in college and one in the Navy. This was a middle-class, African American family that had come to a point in its development in which everyone seemed to be going off in separate directions.

Derrick's mother was a 54-year-old woman who had worked hard most of her life at her civil service job while raising her four children. She was very involved in her church, and after her parents died she had become the matriarch of her family. She had a younger sister who was a single mother and was trying to raise three children. Mrs. C spent a great deal of her time helping her sister. She also helped out with her husband's printing business. Mr. C was a 57-year-old man who had retired from the Navy about 12 years ago. He had worked hard to develop his own business, which had lots of financial problems. Mr. C was rarely at home and spent his time at work or with his friends.

Mr. and Mrs. C were concerned about Derrick's behavior, but both acknowledged that they were tired of raising children. They had worked hard and maintained their responsibilities. They were helping all of their children financially, and felt burdened by this. They expressed a desire to slow things down and spend some time together, and they had been talking about wanting a less hectic lifestyle. Mr. C wanted to sell his business and move to Arizona. Derrick wasn't sure where he fit into the picture; he felt his parents really didn't care what he did, as long as he stayed out of trouble. He said that he got very little attention from them and "that's okay, they don't really know what I'm doing." Mrs. C expressed a lot of concern and frustration with the situation but didn't know what to do. She said she just didn't have the energy to deal with Derrick.

Derrick's difficulties seemed symptomatic of his confusion over recent changes and his perceived lack of security in the family. There was a considerable difference in needs and priorities between Derrick and his parents. They readily admitted that they couldn't keep up with him. Derrick's difficulties in school, marijuana use, and staying out at night could be seen as a cry for attention from his parents and a request for help. Therapy initially needed to validate each family member's position and utilize their concern for each other as an effective motivation to effect some change. Normalizing their situation given their differing needs and developmental stage was also important.

Transformations

Precisely when adolescence begins and ends is open to debate. But one of the most clearly pronounced signs of its beginning is the development of the physical capacity to procreate. Secondary sex characteristics overtly signal this transition, and social definitions become more sexually oriented. Children here can grasp ideas and concepts beyond their own concrete experience, that is, they are able to think more abstractly, although this capacity is measured in different ways across cultures. On the social–emotional front, teenagers struggle with self-definition. They "try on" roles, like trying on jeans at a department store, in order to find the right fit. Without this process, individuals become confused about who they are in life. Parental overreaction to this natural developmental stage can stigmatize a child as "a problem" and lead the adolescent to retreat from family connections. Underreactions, too, can hinder this stage, leaving nonfamily agencies such as the school or police to provide the only limit setting for the adolescent.

Therapists attempt to balance the family need for maintaining structure with the transformational needs of launching an adolescent member. This balance is aided, in part, when the therapist manages the IP label appropriately, creates a metaphor or ritual to capture the family's evolution, and is flexible in responding to the peculiarities of the family.

For example, a 17-year-old adolescent and his family came to therapy with the presenting problem of his drug use. The boy had been experimenting with various drugs and his schoolwork had declined. The family focused on his son's problems so intently that everything seemed to revolve around or about him—who or who did not do the chores, fights between siblings, and conflict between the parents. The therapist created a family sculpt exercise in order to show the family its developmental dilemma. She first asked the client to sit in a chair in the middle of the therapy room and asked each family member to stand in emotional proximity to him. A closely connected "huddle" resulted. She then removed the son from the middle and stated that she was going to work with him on his issues, and then asked the rest of the family to stand where they would like to be in the family. Confusion resulted. The family members looked lost, unable to glimpse a vision of life without the IP's presence. Debriefing following the session evoked important and unacknowledged emotions from various family members about the "positive" function the client served for the family. The family had become developmentally stuck and unable to move forward because of their fears of separateness and individuality.

Most commonly, teenagers are brought to therapy to be "fixed" by the therapist. Although the rest of the family members acknowledge, at some level, that they impact the adolescent, often the focus is "teen versus the family system." Family therapists do well to bring up the complexities of this developmental stage with the family. Psychoeducation helps the family broaden its frame of reference and normalizes the anxiety for everyone. "How are we going to help this child become an adult?" is a useful question to be presented to the entire family. Probing how the parents went through this stage can elicit normalizing information not discussed by the family previously. Having parents describe what their own parents did well or poorly during this stage provokes some systemic reflection.

The therapist should keep in mind, however, that the family isn't the only important concern during this stage. If an adolescent has been displaying addictive patterns, relationships outside of the family might be affecting the teen, and may involve drug use or sexual activity. When the therapist thinks about multiple systems rather than family systems alone, other factors are seen as important to therapeutic work. Referral to a chemical dependency program or inviting friends into therapy might be helpful in managing these important influences. Creatively engaging people from within and without the family to understand the presenting problem assists in solid clinical treatment.

Most civilizations have heralded the passage from childhood to adulthood. Western culture, however, is generally bereft of meaningful ways to mark this transition. Perhaps the most significant ritual for teens in the

United States is acquiring a driver's license. Therapists have found that bringing a ritual into the therapeutic process can assist in creating second-order change (Imber-Black, 1988). Rituals can awaken family members to respond in new ways. One therapist assigned a family the task of creating a "birthday ritual" for each quarter, half, and full year birthday beginning at age 15 and ending at age 18. Using these "birthdays" as points for change, the family negotiated one new privilege for their daughter and one new responsibility. The parents and teenager talked about ways in which they needed to both offer more adulthood status and show more adulthood behavior. Issues such as curfew, driving, chores, allowance, and other areas were "ritually" discussed on these dates until a mutual agreement was found. A celebration of adulthood was prescribed for her 18th birthday.

As so often happens, therapist and clients are challenged by the same things during therapy. Families with adolescents need to be flexible, and so does the therapist. Therapists encounter teenagers who may angrily sulk during most sessions and then suddenly rage at everyone. Parents of teenagers may present as flexible, yet undermine any new suggestions developed during therapy.

Therapists need to keep in mind their "window of opportunity" to influence a family positively. Settling into a long-term therapy posture probably won't fit the needs of the family. Even a weekly therapy schedule might need to be reevaluated. Working with various subsystems of the family, as with very young children, can be quite valuable. Encouraging adolescents to do reverse role-plays (in which the teen plays the parent) or to write poems and letters to express their feelings to the family might enhance therapy, too.

Maintaining a balance between structural expectations (regarding physical safety or time together) and flexibility around the presenting concerns helps develop a strong therapeutic alliance and will model to the family what they need to be doing in their home as well.

Launching Children and Later Life

Issues around launching children and experiencing later life become more prominent as economic instability and life expectancy increase. Families are challenged to accept multiple comings and goings in the family system's membership. In-laws, grandchildren, returning divorced children, aging parents, and death must be accommodated during this life stage. Couples often shift into a dyadic relationship for the first time in life, and are challenged to create a non-child-oriented relationship. Adolescents grow into adults who have their own children, and shift from parent–child to adult–adult connections. Disease, retirement, or disability challenge the family's resources at many turns. Additions and losses pervade the emotional terrain.

Family therapists can act as consultants during this stage. Often a request for a few brief sessions to "sort out what to do next" becomes the therapist's job: "Shall I kick out my 27-year-old cocaine-addicted son from my home?" "Shall we bring Grandma in to live with us after her stroke?" "I thought I was going to have time to travel with my husband, but now we're helping to raise my grandchildren while my daughter works—I'm not sure I want this, but I feel guilty saying that."

We are in changing societal times with few clear directives on how to handle these complex and emotionally charged issues. Each family needs to redefine itself in response to its unique set of beliefs, structural framework, and emotional capacity.

Physically, most people "peak" in their strength and agility during this stage and then move toward progressive deterioration. Particularly for those who have defined themselves in physical terms (attractive, athletic), this stage requires new adjustment around one's self-concept.

Ultimately, personal and relational functioning is connected to the extent of physiological decline. In a culture that encourages independence and celebrates youth, attention to physical decline becomes pronounced in later years. Along with physical concerns, cognitive abilities may be affected by aging. Although people maintain a high ability to continue to learn, new information may be processed more slowly. Memory and reaction time can be impaired, and a small but significant number of people are seriously impacted by dementia and Alzheimer's disease. Caretaking by family member continues to be the key resource for those affected by aging difficulties.

Social–emotional needs of those being launched from a family include the development of intimate relationships and some sort of generativity in the world. Friends and lovers must be found and relationships established. Often individuals seek therapy when limited in this important developmental domain. Being able to use one's gifts, abilities, and interests for the benefit of self and others takes on a prominent focus. Having at least some degree of financial independence from one's family seems to be a part of the process. If these needs aren't met, people experience isolation and stagnation. Often it is in midlife that these concerns are recycled and reviewed once again, although losing one's job or suffering a business failure elicits reassessment, too.

Later in life, social–emotional needs involve reviewing one's life choices and evaluating whether or not one feels integrated regarding what has been accomplished. Peer relationships continue to be a vital connection to good health, although family contacts are important in emergencies. Solid friendships in later years promote well-being at many levels. Gender concerns reemerge as one reviews personal and professional connections. Some men in our culture feel too separated from family connections, while women ponder if they could have been something more than they were. In either case, a life review in connection with continuing family and friendship ties enhances relationships between all members.

Helping clients access resources and deal with grief are important skills a therapist can apply when working with families in launching and later-life stages. Although useful throughout the lifespan, knowledge of community and extended family resources can be critical during these periods. The therapist can encourage the family to use some of its own resources and utilize community resources in achieving positive adjustment for the entire family. Financial, emotional, and practical information can be provided that helps ease some of the strains of this stage. Two cases illustrate these points.

John, age 20, began to have difficulties while away at college. A history major, he had dreams of becoming a lawyer after he finished college. He began drinking heavily during his junior year, and his friends reported to his family that he was acting a bit odd at times. On one occasion, he jumped down a long flight of stairs screaming that the "monkeys were trying to bite me." Hospitalization for a broken ankle and for his first schizophrenic episode followed. John took a leave of absence from college, never to return. When he went home, however, his family found it difficult to cope with him.

Martha, age 78, lived alone after the death of her husband 10 years previously. She lived independently, enjoyed her friends, and gardened and walked each day. One day, her daughter called her several times and did not reach her—an unusual experience. A friend was asked to check on her, and she found Martha unconscious on the floor. Taken to the hospital immediately, Martha was diagnosed with a small cerebral hemorrhage that disabled her permanently. She was unable to walk independently, and thus could no longer live alone or take care of herself. The family faced the decision of what to do next.

In each of these two cases, a family therapist may be included in this decision-making process. The therapist will need to assess the resources of the family as well as the values they hold regarding care for their ill relatives. Broadening support to extended family and friends may be encouraged by the therapist. Also, he or she may be able to access important community resources for the family and assist them in learning to network. Medical specialists, funding sources, self-help and support groups, board and care homes, transitional housing options, respite care, and practical nursing can be invaluable resources for the family.

Therapists who have difficulty managing grief issues would not be well suited for work with families in these stages of the life cycle. Developmentally, the family needs to go through various processes in order to manage either the symbolic or actual death of its members. These include the following:

1. Shared acknowledgment of the death or loss—someone is "gone."
2. Shared expressions of the range of emotions—allow for variations.
3. Reorganization of the family system to accommodate loss—the practical ability for the family to continue to function.
4. Reinvestment into a future life direction without the loved one—finding new ways to continue a meaningful life.

Therapists must assess whether or not the family has gone through each of these stages and can facilitate any unfinished dimensions of the grief.

SPECIAL ISSUES WITH DIVORCING AND REMARRIED FAMILIES

Family adjustment to divorce and remarriage comprises additional stages in the family life cycle—stages that are almost normative in a society where divorce and remarriage is so common. Stress occurs at predictable times for divorcing and remarrying families, and the response to the stress influences how members adjust to shifting family compositions. Family therapists need to keep in mind that emotional cutoffs often hinder adjustment and that, even though there are exceptions, having an ongoing relationship between parents and children is usually the best way to proceed.

Ahrons and Rodgers (1987)found divorcing families go through predictable stages, although not necessarily in sequential order:

1. Decision to divorce, usually by one member before the other
2. Family system is told about the impending divorce
3. Actual physical separation
4. System reorganization
5. System stabilization into a new form

Most researchers indicate that it takes 2–3 years to go through these phases. Successful postdivorce families may often look like the following:

Single parent

- Maintains parental contact with ex-spouse.
- Supports contact of children with ex-spouse and his or her family.
- Rebuilds own social network.

Noncustodial parent

- Maintains parental contact and supports custodial parent's relationship with children.
- Establishes effective parenting relationship with children.
- Rebuilds own social network.

However, research also indicates that only about half of divorcing families are able to develop cooperative coparenting arrangements. The other half of divorced parents continue to fight with their "ex" over the children or neglect this continuing aspect of their relationship. Family therapists often see the emotional fallout on the children from these negative experiences.

Remarried families go through additional stages of the family life cycle. Besides weathering normative transitions and those involving the divorce and any single parenting, these families must negotiate what it means to be "family" on an ongoing basis. Therapists recognize that many remarried families haven't first gone through the earlier stages and therefore enter the remarried transition with many tasks undone. The following case illustrates some of the problems encountered by stepfamilies.

Mr. and Mrs. A presented with arguing and disagreements over raising their two boys. They were a recently married couple, and each spouse had an 11-year-old boy. Most of the couple's other disagreements seem to be resolvable, but discussions involving the boys would quickly escalate, with Mr. A becoming very rigid and angry, and Mrs. A crying and feeling attacked and hopeless. Both partners accused the other of being overly protective of his or her own child. The husband's response to the conflict was to become openly angry, raise his voice, and become opinionated and a bit self-righteous. The wife would cry, withdraw, and say that she had never been talked to like this before. Both agreed that if this problem was not resolved they could not stay married. Mr. A threatened to leave if his wife wouldn't change. There was no indication of physical violence and very little alcohol use.

The husband was a 42-year-old insurance adjuster, retired Navy officer, and Vietnam veteran. He was 21 years old when he married for the first time. That marriage lasted for 3 years, and he was not sure why it ended. His son was born during his second marriage, which lasted 6 years. That relationship ended because his wife started seeing other men. He described his ex-wife as irresponsible and childlike. His son had occasional contact with her. Mr. A's family of origin was described as a "good learning experience." His father was a career Marine officer and his mother was a homemaker. His parents' marriage was described as tumultuous. They divorced when he was 14.

Mr. A was a very committed and concerned father who was very close to his son. He was a proud man who spoke directly and expressed his opinions freely. He was involved with his son in sports and his schoolwork, and they liked to travel together. His son was a good student, well mannered, and an excellent athlete.

Mrs. A was a 40-year-old physical therapist. She had been married for 12 years; her husband had died abruptly of a heart attack about 3 years earlier. He was 40 years old at the time. She cared for him very much and described him as "sensitive, caring, easy to get along with, but a bit boring." She came from a very religious, conservative, stable family environment. Her parents were happily married and had been supportive throughout her marriage and since the death of her husband. She described herself as easy-going, sensitive, and emotional. She was very close to her son and felt bad that he lost his father. Her son was bright, conservative, and did well in school. He was not particularly good at sports but excelled in math, science, and computers.

Mr. A had some negative feelings about therapy. He went with his ex-wife and had found it of little value. Mrs. A was afraid that without help they would likely get a divorce because of the fights and Mr. A's primary allegiance to his son. Mrs. A said, "We just can't agree about anything the boys do, and the smallest thing turns into a major battle every time."

This case demonstrates that stepfamilies do not, and cannot, come together as biological families do. Allegiances between biological parent and child remain strong, and in the early going, need to be protected. Rather than be forced into the mold of the biological family, stepfamilies and the therapists who treat them can benefit from an understanding of the various stages of stepfamily formation:

1. Entering a new relationship—recovery from the losses of the first marriage or adequate "emotional divorce" is explored.
2. Conceptualizing and planning the new marriage and family—time and patience are needed for adjustment to the ambiguity and complexity of the new family; fears, loyalty conflicts, and system membership are focal, while ex-spouses work out a cooperative coparental relationship; multiple new roles, affective issues, and boundaries are negotiated.
3. Remarriage and family reconstitution—involves final resolution of the attachment to one's previous spouse and the "ideal" intact

family, and acceptance of a different model of family with permeable boundaries.

Family therapists need to recognize their strengths and limitations when assisting families through these developmental stages. At a time when social transitions are complex and abundant, it is impossible to provide a single model of family that fits everyone. Rather, we come alongside families to help them invent a new form of family structure that will work for them.

Divorce and remarriage almost always involves some level of conflict. Substantive research affirms again and again that children exposed to continuing parental conflict are negatively affected. Individuals and families will not be able to move beyond their presenting problems unless they can manage conflict constructively. Therapists must advise and set limits on the amount of conflict permitted within the family.

In addition, therapists must determine how able a family is to operate in a coparenting relationship. When parents are unable to cooperate for the sake of their children, therapists must consider how to define relationships between parents and children separately. Complete cutoff with a parent might occur, but should not be an acceptable solution for the family. Finding creative ways to have some continuing contact with a noncustodial parents will help everyone.

Therapists should guard against colluding with particular family members because doing so can closes off relationships that might be therapeutic. For example, a mother might say that her ex-husband has "no interest" in their difficult teenage daughter. If you contact the father, however, you may find he does have interest and can assist the family and support his ex-wife in the parenting the teen. Each case regarding connections with noncustodial parents needs to be considered carefully.

Some newly formed relationships sound too good to be true—and they are. People who were hurt in former relationships are often blind to the inherent difficulties and differences between new partners. Encouraging the expression of differences and practically exploring possible problems for the family encourages true mutuality.

Often extended family—aunts, uncles, grandparents, and cousins— had significant relationships severed as a result of divorce. These relatives can often function as family resources during difficult transitional stages. Therapists should ask about these people and encourage contact when appropriate.

Families recovering from divorce and those forming stepfamilies need approximately 2 years to go through each developmental process. It's important to remind families that it takes time and patience to negotiate these stages successfully. Some don't manage well because of the continuing battles between family members. Noticing and encouraging successful developmental steps and normalizing struggles will help families use their resources to the fullest.

MEDIATION AND CHILD CUSTODY EVALUATION

Family therapists have become an important resource to the legal system in determining the separating and postdivorce world of the family. Many states require families to work with family court mediators, a large number of whom have family therapy training, to assist a family in negotiating divorce and custody settlements. Mediators have helped to relieve our overburdened court system in many states. Specialized training allows mediators to become an important link between the legal and family systems.

Most state's legal systems have moved from the "tender years doctrine" of generally awarding mothers custody to a "best interests of the child" standard. The Uniform Marriage and Divorce Act (Bureau of National Affairs, Inc., 1982) offers these guidelines in Section 402:

> The court shall determined custody in accordance with the best interest of the child. The court shall consider all relevant factors, including:
>
> 1. the wishes of the child's parent or parents as to his custody;
> 2. the wishes of the child as to his custodian;
> 3. the interaction and interrelationship of the child with his parent or parents, his siblings, an any other person who may significantly affect the child's best interest;
> 4. the child's adjustment to his home, school, and community; and
> 5. the mental and physical health of all individuals involved.
>
> The court shall not consider conduct of a proposed custodian that does not affect his relationship to the child.

Judges often rely on the advice of experts to determine the "best interests" standard; this relational information can be obtained from a family therapist's observations and opinions. Parents as well as the court can seek the services of family therapists for this purpose. Sometimes interns and therapists are surprised to discover the "true" motive for a person seeking therapy after it has been going on for awhile—the client requests a letter or report from the therapist to be used in a divorce court or custody proceeding.

Therapists need to be informed about the divorce and custody laws of their state in order to work competently in this arena. If one wants to learn how to do custody evaluations, it is best to be mentored by someone who has done them over several years and is recognized by the court.

Therapists need to be aware of the research outcomes regarding high-conflict divorce. Finally, therapists need a clear contract regarding their role in any divorce or custody case. Often, it's best to be hired as an expert to the court rather than be triangulated into serving as an expert for one parent against the other parent. Family therapists have much to contribute to the legal–family interface in the years to come.

SPECIAL ISSUES WITH SINGLE-PARENT POOR FAMILIES

The family life cycle stages discussed in this chapter are based on a middle-class paradigm. Things are different for poor, single-parent families—social and economic realities are the drivers behind a different set of life cycle stages.

Colon (1980) sees the family life cycle of the poor as having three phases:

1. The unattached young adult (who may actually be 11 or 12 years old)—on his or her own and virtually unaccountable to adults.
2. Families with children—a phase that occupies most of the lifespan and commonly has a three-generation household.
3. The nonevolved grandmother—still involved in a central role in old age, still actively in charge of the generations below her.

Aponte (1976) and Minuchin et al. (1967) offer clinical approaches to working with single-parent poor families: structurally defining parental roles when parents, live-in partners, and grandparents have a say about the household children; encouraging the development of the biological mother's personal resources; and increasing access to more social and economic resources. The following case provides a glimpse of what life can be like for clients who are single mothers living in poverty, as well as some appropriate interventions.

Ms. G was a single mother who was raising three children: 7-year-old Eloisa, 10-year-old Juan, and 13-year-old Gilbert. Ms. G's husband had left the family when Eloisa was 2 years old, and he had provided no support and had no contact with the children. This Hispanic family lived in a small two-bedroom apartment. The mother worked long hours cleaning houses, and she had little money to pay for anything but the bare essentials. Her long hours made supervision of the children difficult, so she often left Gilbert in charge. This became an increasingly difficult situation because he resented the responsibility and would leave his brother and sister alone for long periods.

Ms. G sought counseling at the recommendation of the school counselor. Gilbert had become a "behavior problem" at school. Since entering junior high school a year and a half before, he began cutting classes and showing little interest in his school work. His mother said that he was hanging out with "gang bangers," but she didn't think that Gilbert was involved in a gang. She had tried to get his uncle to spend time with Gilbert but his work schedule made this difficult. Gilbert seemed angry with and disappointed by any authority figures. His grades kept dropping and his teachers had added Saturday school as a steady part of his weekly routine.

Ms. G felt frustrated and helpless in trying to handle Gilbert. She said she was almost ready to give up and concentrate on the younger ones. She couldn't afford to pay for childcare after school and so had begun to send the younger children to the local Boys and Girls Club, but she was afraid of the effects that the older neighborhood children would have on Juan and Eloisa.

Ms. G had been receiving some help from her mother until they began having difficulties about 2 years earlier. Ms. G had begun dating a man that her mother disliked, and this caused considerable conflict between the two women. The children's grandmother wanted to maintain contact with them but, Ms. G's anger and resentment caused her to severely limit their visits.

Ms. G's lack of financial resources and emotional support was quite apparent. The therapist's job was to assist her in making effective use of community resources and in considering family therapy that includes the children, Ms. G, and her mother. Single parents like Ms. G often lack the time and energy to make use of community resources and feel overwhelmed in attempting to maintain all of their responsibilities. Providing support and identifying outside resources is an essential element in working with this type of case.

While single-parent families often face daunting problems, many of them are competent and successful. Lindblad-Goldberg (1989) has identified successful single-parent families as those in which parents, usually mothers, showed less depression, experienced more control over their lives, displayed more effective executive authority with their children, launched their older children from the household, communicated more effectively, developed close family ties, cognitively highlighted positive life experiences rather than negative ones, and utilized social networks creatively.

The expertise of family therapists is the family. Knowledge of the family's lifespan and the presenting problems associated with each developmental stage assists us in providing solid clinical work.

8

Working with Couples

Mary is a 29-year-old Caucasian woman who has been recovering from alcoholism for the past year. Bob is a 32-year-old Caucasian male who is also recovering from alcoholism. Bob is being treated for depression by a psychiatrist who is prescribing Prozac for him. Mary has been to two individual therapists through her health maintenance organization, but feels dissatisfied with them because they don't really understand "the disease" of alcoholism.

This couple has been living together for the past 6 years. They have separated several times during that period. They were married 1 year ago. Bob says that he is increasingly unhappy in the marriage and has decided that he wants a separation. Mary has said that she "can't stand the thought of being without him" and wants to keep the relationship together. She reports "always feeling insecure" and doubting herself. She feels very confused by Bob's "double messages" because he says he wants a divorce but continues to act friendly and interested in Mary. He invites her to do things with him and desires to be with her sexually. He also tells Mary that he doesn't love her any more. They argue and bicker about lots of little things, but seem able to discuss important concerns. Still, many conflicts go unresolved.

Mary is requesting couple therapy to "try to either resolve these issues or get some closure." Bob is reluctant to go to therapy but has indicated that he will try it for one or two visits. They saw a couple therapist previously but didn't continue, as Mary felt that the therapist sided with Bob, and didn't really understand the situation.

This case presents a complex web of symptoms and concerns. The individual issues include the alcoholism, Bob's depression, and Mary's low self-esteem. The couple's issues include their confusion about whether to stay together or not, their inability to resolve conflict, and their poor communication. The case is complicated by their previous, unsatisfactory attempt at therapy.

How does a therapist understand and work with such a couple? This chapter focuses on couples who seek help for their continuing relationship. We explain the two key systemic lessons needed for beginning (and probably all) therapists to do effective couple therapy. We then move to common dynamics and problems presented by couples and suggest ways to understand and deal with them.

KEYS TO PROVIDING SOLID COUPLE THERAPY

What makes a good couple therapist? Therapists in training seem to either love or hate couple work. Could there be a reason? A new intern, in commenting about her first couple session, said, "I felt beat up, totally stuck in the middle. Anytime I tried to listen to the husband, the wife interrupted and told me her version. I didn't know what to do."

Key Number 1

Effective couple therapists must have the ability to manage a three-person relationship. The therapist literally becomes the emotional and relational hub for the couples' interactions, and can provide the foundation for solid couples work, depending on how well he or she works with a triangle, or three-person relationship.

Family systems and other sociological theories focus on the various ways the presence of a third person can impact a dyadic relationship. Just think of how awkward you feel when you go up to two friends who seem to be having a private conversation and you begin to notice the interactional changes that occur simply by your added presence. Structural family therapy clearly describes how children are triangulated into a conflictual marital relationship to diffuse the intensity of the couple's relationship. A third party (such as a therapist) can enhance or detract (as does an affair) from the couple's relationship.

Key Number 2

The primary developmental task for couples is to create a new system. Most important here is the word "new." Partnering is a process in which each person brings into the relationship his or her history and personal attributes and attempts to combine them with another's, so that a new system emerges. Couples commonly come for counseling when their attempts to create this new system fail. Of course, societal and cultural expectations strongly influence this very personal process, too.

Different couple therapies highlight particular aspects of this failed developmental process. Behavioral therapies emphasize common content areas in which couples bog down (finances, sex, children) and teach team-building skills. Solution-focused therapy ferrets out times when the couple did act as a team. Experiential therapies and more recent experiential/strategic approaches such as emotionally focused therapy help to create times when the couple "feels" like a couple.

In this chapter we will deal mostly with conjoint couple counseling and not with group therapy with couples, although the latter is a very important treatment approach. Groups are helpful because they normalize the difficulties and model the work it takes to create a new system. Couples' groups help participants to recognize that partnering is done throughout the lifespan, and that certain skills must be in place to develop a functioning unit. Although many family therapists will not have the opportunity to provide group therapy, they will do conjoint couple therapy.

CREATING A THERAPEUTIC TRIANGLE

Keeping in mind the goal of creating a therapeutic triangle in order to form a new system, therapists can connect to the couple in several ways, as shown in Figure 8.1A–C.

Empathizing with Individuals

In Panel A, the therapist attempts to connect empathically with each person. For example, he or she might ask at the beginning of the first session, "What brings you in today and how might you want me to help?" With this, one partner might say, "I'm not happy in my marriage and I haven't been for a long time. I don't know what to do. I've tried but nothing seems to work." The therapist might empathically respond, "So you're sad and frustrated with the way your marriage is right now and you're confused about what to do next." The client responds, "Yes, that's it."

It's important to remember that when the therapist takes an individually empathic position, it impacts the triadic relationship. The partner who is not being attended to experiences being "left out" for a moment. (In Figure 8.1A, only connection 1 or 2 can be engaged.) Often the unattended person will interrupt the process to receive attention or to "correct" the therapist's understanding. (Many psychodynamically oriented therapists

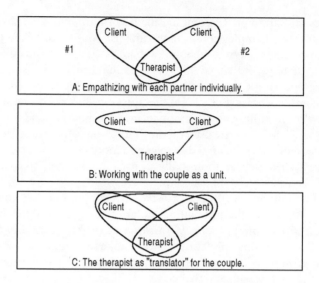

FIGURE 8.1. Therapeutic triangles.

use the "left out" partner's response to help diagnose that person. In addition, the intersubjective experience of the therapist with each partner aids the transference needed for psychodynamic therapy to proceed.) If the therapist allows this interruption to occur repeatedly without taking charge of the interaction, the therapist will begin to feel bumped back and forth between the two individuals, much like a tennis ball between two players.

Beginning therapists often get stuck at this stage. They know how to do individual therapy with each partner, but don't know where to go next. Instead of managing the entire triangle, the therapist only listens to each partner individually during the session. Often the tension between the couple heightens and the interaction becomes more conflictual. Without knowing how to triadically manage the case, the therapist might even recommend each person be seen separately. Although useful at times, most often couple work needs to be done with both partners present. Separating the couple mostly helps the therapist's anxiety, not the couple's.

Especially at the beginning of couple therapy, the therapist can use empathic connection with each partner to create a therapeutic alliance. However, it's wise for the therapist to direct this interaction, to tell the couple that each of them will get their turn, and to emphasize that it's important for the therapist to understand each person's concerns.

Statistics indicate that about 40% of couples don't return for a second session. Why is this? Many beginning therapists don't know how to manage the relationship triangle effectively. The couple experience interactions similar to the ones at home and find therapy a waste of time and money. When the therapist builds the relationship with each person during the first session, then each one usually experiences a beginning bond and trust with the therapist and will want to continue in therapy. Taking this empathic stance with a couple isn't the only position a therapist can take. In order to be effective, the therapist must be able to move fluidly to other positions.

Working with the Couple as a Unit

Behavioral and solution-focused therapists focus on this dimension of couple therapy working with the couple as a unit (Figure 8.1B). Rather than spending much energy on the therapist–client personal relationship, the therapist takes a position of orchestrating new behaviors between the couple. In behavioral therapy, the therapist helps train the couple in new positive communication and conflict resolution skills, often by having the couple engage in active-listening exercises during the session and practice at home. In solution-focused couple work, the therapist promotes better interactions by asking therapeutically minded questions to uncover the couple's own repertoire of "lost" positive behaviors. These positive exceptions are then emphasized by the therapist and given as homework to the couple.

For instance, rather than focusing on the times the couple argued during the past day, the therapist asks the couple instead to describe times when the couple was not arguing and were enjoying each other's company and/or able to make a joint decision harmoniously.

Much of traditional couple therapy, especially any with educational components, takes this triadic stance. Although not often articulated as a core developmental task for the couple, the creation of a new system in which each person can exist without symptoms is assumed by these approaches to be the task of therapy. Skills and positive interactional experiences are needed to create and maintain the new system.

When a beginning therapist is unsure of how to proceed when doing work with a couple or when a couple negatively escalates their interaction, the therapist can interrupt the process by restating the powerful assumption of this triadic position: For example, "What we're trying to do here is create a new kind of relationship where both of your concerns and needs can be honored. Rather than living together as opponents, let's work on being on the same team." Another comment from this perspective might be "We all know that partnering is hard work. In many ways, you've never been 'married' on this issue and this is the first time you're trying to find a really useful way to work it out." These kind of comments often lessen the tension between the couple since both are joined in wanting to make the relationship work. If this doesn't calm them, it may mean that at least one person has already left the relationship and has given up attempting to be a partner. Alternatively, a lack of calming might indicate the therapist's return to the previously discussed "empathic" position with respect to one of the partners. In such a case, the therapist should attend to and possibly reengage the other person.

The Therapist as "Translator" for the Couple

A final triadic position the therapist can take to manage couple therapy effectively is that of an interpreter or translator (Figure 8.1C). In this focus, the therapist functions as one who understands that each partner's behaviors, perceptions, and experiences influence the couple's functioning. The therapist creates new ways for the couple to understand each other, often taking a mediating position. For example, couples commonly battle with each other because each person is trying to re-create his or her family of origin in the new family. Part of what creates a new system are interactions that respect some combination of each person's history and values. Without this new system perspective, the couple continues to fight.

For example, a young couple comes in with complaints about how they are spending their money. One partner came from a structured family where money was carefully accounted for, while the other partner's family allowed each individual to spend as they wished. Each partner argues for his or her own "right way" to oversee the family budget and criticizes the other for being either "tight" or irresponsible. The therapist can first acknowledge the strengths and possible liabilities of each person's family of origin lessons about money. Then he or she might reframe the couple's battle as "very healthy—each person has a different expertise that can benefit the relationship and both need to be heard." Then the therapist can wonder out loud if the couple might find a way to embrace each other's expertise, and, in so doing, strengthen the marriage. In this way the therapist first translates, then mediates, for the couple.

Basic to understanding this systemic position is the assumption that partnering requires a recognition that each person is different in some way. These differences will either promote a healthy, differentiated system or will disintegrate into a "power play" wherein each partner wants to win control of the relationship. The therapist, rather than taking sides, promotes a relationship based on the unit of the couple rather than on each person individually. The therapist simultaneously translates and verbalizes how each partner brings into the relationship different ways of being and doing.

Some Bowenian-based approaches take this position in providing couple therapy. A therapy session might look like this: Each partner reviews his or her family of origin using the genogram. The therapist facilitates a discussion about the interpersonal patterns shown from the family and explores whether or not these patterns are present in the couple's relationship. The therapist might ask whether or not the other partner also notices any patterns, and inquires of either or both partners which patterns should be kept and which should be changed in their new relationship. In this way, the couple learns how their own difficulties are tied to previous family of origin difficulties. The therapist helps them translate their presenting issues into more understandable and therefore more manageable problems. A stance of differentiation and newness is taken.

Simply stated, the more complicated the couple's presenting problems, the more the therapist must actively take all three of the systemic positions reviewed here. When a less complicated case appears, the therapist can select which of the three positions will be most helpful, often moving to the "couple as a unit" stance. Sometimes this choice simply comes from the training one has had ("I know solution-focused therapy"), while at other times the choice can be made with the couple ("We can work on your problems using either behavioral marital therapy or transgenerational therapy").

The following three case studies demonstrate how the various systemic stances might look, both individually and in combination.

Case Study: Stance 2

A couple comes to therapy presenting with fights over parenting and money. The therapist determines several strengths in their relationship and selects a behavioral marital therapy approach with the couple. After developing a list of caring behaviors, the couple works on caring days to increase positive interactions. When areas of common interest are identified, communication and problem-solving skills are practiced. After some criterion of proficiency is met, the therapist directs the couple to address parenting issues first using their new communication skills, and then to work on problem-solving strategies. The couple selects a "noninterruption" policy in front of their children. They also find that spending weekly "fun time" together sets a better tone in their relationship to discuss problematic issues surrounding money.

In this case, the therapist focuses on developing new relationship patterns that address the couple's presenting problems. Individual experiences are less of a focus; the therapist is more goal directed and works with the couple as a unit.

Case Study: Stance 3

A blended family presents with conflict in their marriage. They mostly argue over parenting of the wife's biological children, who live with them about 70% of the time. The husband feels angry about the "flaky, alcoholic" father of the children, who only pays child support intermittently. Sometimes the husband displays angry outbursts toward the children since they seem to be "flaky" too. The wife often finds herself stuck in the middle between the man she loves and her children, whom she feels need to be protected. She also feels it's important for the children to have contact with the biological father. The therapist, who explores transgenerational patterns, notes that the husband grew up with an alcoholic father whom he cut himself off from during his 20s. This pattern seems to be similar to the current agenda for stepfather. The therapist also notes that the wife grew up as the middle child of two sisters. She used to stand up to her mother, who was verbally abusive toward the sisters. She also had a distant but consistent relationship with her own father.

The therapist begins to translate and to connect each partner's current strategy for coping with their current family to their respective family of origin patterns. She works to help each person see his or her own legacies and to explore whether each wishes to continue this strategy. The possibility for new options can also be examined.

Case Study: Stances 1, 2, 3

A couple comes to therapy after 12 years of marriage. The wife recently began to deal with her sexual abuse history. She sometimes has flashbacks of early traumatic memories, which are affecting her sleep. Her sexual interest is very low and there is limited sexual activity in the relationship. Her husband feels he has been patient with her over the past year, but he believes it is time to "move on." There has been more tension in the marriage and both wonder whether or not they can survive together.

The therapist takes time to clearly understand each partner (Stance 1). She explores the affective tone behind the problems (such as fear and abandonment), and begins to explore and translate the issues into new affective information for each partner. Finally, she might encourage each partner to communicate with the other using a deeper affective agenda (Stance 2). This emotionally focused perspective (Greenberg & Johnson, 1988) uses all three stances for its couple therapy.

WHEN COUPLE THERAPY MIGHT NOT WORK

Couple therapy is not always the therapy of choice. Although therapists might differ in how they decide for or against couple work, several indicators point to the limits of conjoint sessions. One might be the individual pathology presented by one of the partners. For example, severe depression, psychotic thought processes, or active alcoholism or drug abuse in one partner, or explosive violence between the couple are potential warning signs that couple therapy might be inappropriate. One way to assess whether presenting problems are conducive to conjoint sessions is to determine if a connection or therapeutic relationship can be made between the therapist and the individual or system. If the therapist fails to develop some structure around the couple's interactions, if one of the pair comes drunk or high to the session, or if an individual's affect so influences the session that it severely hinders any interventions, then the therapist would be wise to separate the couple or refer one or both partners to other resources before embarking on conjoint therapy.

There is wisdom in using individual therapy, or individual group sessions, along with couple therapy. Simultaneously working at an individual and systemic level is merited in complicated cases. The major limits, of course, are the financial and therapeutic resources available for the work to be done. Prioritizing and delineating an overall treatment plan that shows therapy can be provided from different and complementary system levels (biological, individual, relational, cultural) often helps the couple engage in the tough work of therapy.

COMMON PROBLEMS PRESENTED IN COUPLE THERAPY

I'm Right; You're Wrong

Commitment to a new system, the first task of couples forming a family, often brings with it fights surrounding whose personal or family of origin style will prevail. Arguments on topics ranging from the correct way to unroll toilet paper to the place spirituality will take in family life might not be resolved successfully by the couple alone. Some will turn to family therapists for help. As discussed previously, the therapist has some choices as to what stance he or she takes in working with the couple. One helpful position is to work with the couple as a unit, framing their arguments as a very normal developmental problem of forming a common household. The therapist may challenge the couple to make room in their relationship for each other's concerns, so that the relationship can win. Otherwise, the couple stays in a competitive, win–lose pattern that is often de-structive to the relationship in the long run. Skill training and developing rules about listening and decision making can be helpful. Trying out "new mutual attempts" in problem areas and bringing back feedback about the success or failure of these attempts stretch the couple's flexibility. Fur-ther, the therapist can question whether the couple needs to come to reso-lution on all conflictual areas. After understanding each other's position, agreeing to disagree on some topics might provide relief and a new sys-tem model for the couple.

The Escalation Cycle

Parents know that "time-outs" commonly help children when they can no longer manage their feelings well. Adults also need to learn ways to stop and disrupt unhealthy patterns. Research indicates that negative in-teractional patterns tend to continue spiraling, making smaller problems into much larger ones. Behavior therapists for years have utilized many specific cognitive or behavioral interventions to stop and redirect thoughts and behaviors. Couples need to understand their escalation patterns and be given specific methods to stop these destructive sequences, such as time-outs with discussion to be continued later or time-outs that restart the discussion using solid communication techniques.

Pursuer–Distancer

Often one partner appears to take the lead more often in working on the couple's relationship. Frequently this is the woman, since women have been socialized to take care of relationship issues more than men. The pattern that develops when one partner initiates and the other responds by back-ing away is common with many couples who present in therapy. Consider the story of James and Jamie:

Jamie is a 43-year-old Caucasian woman who has been primarily responsible for raising her three children. She works as a teacher, and has had to juggle all of her responsibilities since she began to have kids 13 years ago. James is a 45-year-old businessman who works hard at his job, which involves considerable travel. Jamie has felt responsible for running the household, working, and raising the children. She has felt overwhelmed and stressed by all of the tasks and has looked to James for emotional support. They have been married for 15 years. James has been unavail-able much of that time. Jamie's requests for support and time are often met with anger from James. He feels that his wife doesn't understand how hard he works, and that when he gets home he wants to be left alone to recover. Jamie's pursuit of time alone with James is often met by his withdrawal and by his working on the computer. He says he wants to do things together, but when he feels ready—not when he feels pushed. The more Jamie pushes James, the more he seems to pull away.

Labeling this interactional sequence for the couple can begin the change process. Celebrating the fact that the distancing partner has come to therapy (which is a nondistancing move) is a reminder of the potential for new patterns to be established. Reframing for the couple that men and women handle conflict differently also helps. Longitudinal research on marriage shows that some couples manage relationship conflict well, with one partner productively bringing up relationship problems and one who listens and talks, rather than avoiding discussion or shutting down.

Pursuer–distancer patterns can be challenged when a couple agrees to try the new ways of communicating that are offered in therapy.

Unmet Needs and Other Issues from the Past

Powerful emotions are often presented to the therapist, some of which may be connected to one or both of the partners' personal histories. For example, a husband's loud voice may trigger memories of the wife's emotional and physical abuse as a child. The therapist must determine how much historical information is necessary for the partners to work together. Unique to most systemically oriented therapists is the commitment to working on history as it is presented currently in the couple's relationship. For example, object relations family therapy identifies the powerful tie of a person's present feelings to unmet self-development needs of earlier life. People who work with couples recognize that individuals don't fall in love with just anyone, but with people who are, in some way, tied to the dynamics of earlier familial and relational experiences. However, although some couples come to therapy expecting to review and explore their psychodynamic past, others just want to be fixed now. Matching the type of therapy to the couple's agenda helps clarify the matter of history.

Beginning therapists often feel confused themselves about how the past influences the present and how much of the past needs to be explored in order to do solid clinical work. The therapist must continue to reflect, read, and try out different therapeutic strategies with couples in order to answer this question. It is an important issue for those doing couple work, and the answers you find will probably change over the course of your career.

Ambivalence

One or both partners may come to couple counseling with mixed and confused feelings and thoughts. A person might simultaneously hold the belief that it would be wise to end the relationship and the belief that there's still hope for change. Therapists need to understand and reflect back this ambivalence to clients, and not push therapy too far ahead. Solid pacing (discussed in Chapter 7) is essential. Ambivalence may be managed by normalizing it and by setting up very short-term goals. Setting up two or three therapy sessions to explore whether or not change is possible can be helpful as well. Prematurely deciding to end or to work on salvaging the relationship often aligns the therapist with only one partner. The therapist can take a neutral, exploratory stance that looks at the issues attached to the ambivalent partner's perspective. With this posture, the therapist might move the couple to decide on some goals together.

LONGITUDINAL RESEARCH ON COUPLES

Marriage and family therapies are often criticized for their lack of empirical support. In fact, some therapists make a distinction between "marital counseling" and "family therapy" because of the bias against viewing marital counseling as a valid treatment, a bias reflected in legislative and payer organizations' (private insurance and health maintenance organizations) unwillingness to pay for marital therapy. The growing focus on funding treatment only for "medically necessary conditions" such as DSM-IV mental disorders precludes funding for marital counseling. Instead, marital counseling is viewed as a less valid, less effective treatment than other types of therapy (*Consumer Reports*, 1995).

This distinction between marital and other types of therapy is unfortunate and ironic. In fact, behavioral marital therapies have some of the most impressive empirical support for efficacy of all types of therapies (Sanderson, 1995). Researchers talk in terms of the ability to predict a phenomenon as one of the hallmark qualities of the scientific method. John Gottman, a seminal marital researcher, has developed a model that enables him to predict with 98% accuracy which couples will eventually divorce, simply by watching them interact over a conflict area.

Marital therapy has proven to be highly effective in treating depressed spouses (Clarkin, Haas, & Glick, 1988; Prince & Jacobson, 1995a). If therapists and payers genuinely support a biopsychosocial model, marital therapy should be a viable treatment—even for many mental disorders. Marital therapy is currently being explored as a treatment for mood and anxiety disorders, but it will be several years before results are known.

Behavioral marital researchers focus on how couples resolve conflict in order to predict divorce. Table 8.1 uses both researchers' and couples' experiences in its illustration of risk factors related to marital distress.

TABLE 8.1. Possible Predictors of Current and Future Marital Problems

Research findings

1. Rapid escalation of negative emotions—especially anger (this may or may not lead to violence).
2. Inability to successfully exit out of a heated argument.
3. Positive behaviors of one partner are contingent upon positive behaviors of the other partner.
4. During interactions, partners feel negative or neutral about each other's statements rather than positive. Over time, this unrewarding communication leads to distance and withdrawal.
5. When one partner responds more negatively to a statement than the other partner intended.
6. Blaming partner for marital problems and feeling that partner (vs. self) must change for relationship to improve.
7. High physiological arousal (getting very heated) even when thinking about talking to each other.
8. Pattern of making decisions that put self or other interest above the relationship.
9. Not feeling confident that when problems arise they can be solved.

Couples' experiences

1. When fighting, you attack each other or one person attacks and the other defends, as compared to listening to each other's gripes.
2. One partner says that more sex will lead to greater closeness and the other partner says that more closeness will lead to more sex.
3. When one partner (in many marriages, the wife) wants to sit down and talk (and be close) and the other (in many marriages, the husband) feels that a fight will soon ensue.
4. Knowing what a fight will be like, how it will end, feeling "here we go again," and then having the fight anyway.
5. Inability to reach satisfying agreements on issues all couples encounter at various stages of the family life cycle (e.g., having children, how to raise children, career decisions).
6. Decrease in time spent together—especially talking face-to-face with no disturbances (e.g., television).
7. Decrease in fun times together.
8. Feeling that you are not listening to your partner and are not listened to by your partner.
9. Feeling taken for granted or that you are taking your spouse for granted.
10. Feeling that things won't change in the relationship.

Note. From Markman (1987).

While Leber, St. Peters, and Markman (1996) point out that 70% of couples' conflicts don't need specific resolution, responses to these conflicts can effectively destroy a marriage. Most behavioral marital researchers agree that there needs to be a 5:1 ratio of positive to negative interactions for couples to view their marriage as satisfying. As long as the relationship is going smoothly, couples take their commitment to each other for granted. However, when negative interactions such as destructive fighting increases, couples can begin to question their commitment to the relationship.

Perhaps most couples understand the potentially corrosive effects of conflict because couples vary in their "conflict style" (Gottman, 1994). Volatile couples frequently engage in intense marital conflict but have equally positive and passionate interactions. Validating couples—those who focus on the friendship qualities of their marriage—are willing to fight but do so less frequently and less intensely. Partners in conflict-avoiding marriages are uncomfortable with overt expression of anger, and they avoid conflict altogether. These couples usually have traditional gender-role division in their marriages and focus on the functional and societal reasons for being married rather than on the closeness of the relationship. Hostile and hostile–detached marriages are those moving toward marital deterioration. Gottman (1994) suggests that marital therapists vary the type of therapy they do depending on the couple's typical response to conflict. Most "problem-solving" models for couple therapy that are popular today only fit the validating type of couple.

Qualities about the conflict process that are especially corrosive include criticism, contempt, defensiveness, and stonewalling. These same factors are some of the keynote signatures of divorce. If a therapist observes a couple in which a potential conflict quickly escalates, with the wife displaying contempt and disgust toward her husband and the husband responding defensively, whining, distancing, and stonewalling, the therapist can know the couple is at risk of emotional or legal divorce.

After years of repeating the same negative escalation cycles, both partners can feel flooded or overwhelmed by their own emotions and those of their partner. This feeling can result in a high level of physiological arousal that is aversive. In order to avoid these painful emotional and physical situations, a spouse may distance. The couple begins to view their problems as severe, and each partner decides that it's best to work out problems alone. While each feels lonely, the couple also begin to live "parallel lives." In essence, the emotional divorce takes place before the physical or legal divorce. Not every couple living parallel lives actually divorces. Instead, partners may decide to remain legally married but end their emotional connection. Gottman summarizes his ideas about marriage by saying "the path to improving a relationship over time lies in feeling safe, even when handling disagreement, which . . . concerns feeling loved and respected" (quoted in Patterson, 1990, p. 96). This view suggests that the couple must learn how each partner may bring up areas of potential conflict without eliciting a defensive, stubborn, whining response. Spouses must stay engaged in the discussion, watch for escalation of negative emotion, and communicate to their spouses that they're listening and taking the other's comments seriously.

Programs such as the Prevention and Relationship Enhancement Program (PREP) teach couples these skills by covering such techniques as speaker/listener skills, or by scheduling weekly couple meetings. Listening nondefensively, communicating that you are listening and understanding what your spouse is saying (though not necessarily agreeing), and staying calm are three skills that behavioral marital therapists emphasize.

The behavioral marital therapy movement offers a wealth of books, courses, videotapes, and other resources. Clifford Notarius, Howard Markman, and John Gottman have all written books for the public that are based on solid empirical data. Therapists who are comfortable using a cognitive-behavioral approach with a complementary focus on psychoeducation will find ample resources.

A major criticism of cognitive-behavioral therapy is that it ignores emotion, a central quality of any marriage. Indeed, Gottman refers to "hidden agendas" of feeling loved and respected. However, a marital therapy that focuses even more directly on the major influence of emotion is "emotionally focused" therapy, which was developed by Leslie Greenberg and Susan Johnson. Emotionally focused therapy draws on theoretical assumptions from Gestalt therapy, attachment theory, and general systems theory. Emotionally focused therapy has the same empirical support that is found for the behavioral therapies. Greenberg and Johnson (1988)distinguish between primary emotions, such as feeling loved, and secondary emotions that can mask the basic primary emotions. The therapist's task is to uncover the primary emotions influencing each person's behavior during negative interaction cycles. The therapist goes on to help each partner accept his or her disowned needs and those of the partner.

SPECIAL TOPICS

Gender, cultural, and societal factors influence many of the topics discussed next. In a changing world that is full of new challenges, the norms and rules of behavior are less clearly determined and more personally defined. While patterns still exist, they're often unique to individuals. A therapist must act flexibly and intelligently with couples, yet he or she is limited by gender, cultural, and social experiences. Selected for discussion are common couple therapy issues that often elicit strong responses from beginning therapists.

Dealing with Infidelity

Research indicates that women and men participate in and understand extramarital affairs differently. Women tend to engage in emotional relationships while men engage in sexual ones (Brown, 1991). This resonates with other gender patterns that find women tend to associate intimacy with verbal communication while men associate intimacy with shared activities, including sexual relations (Rubin, 1983; Tannen, 1990).

Two components seem evident in infidelity: (1) breaking the couple's agreement regarding sexual and/or emotional exclusivity, and (2) secrecy. A partner might react to an "emotional" affair as strongly as to a "physical" affair. The therapist must understand the couple's relational contract and the meaning of the breach of the contract; therapy could be hindered by not knowing about an affair or "broken contract," or the therapist may be triangulated by one of the partners into keeping the secret from the other.

Many marital therapists don't believe that keeping secrets for very long is clinically or ethically responsible behavior. Some choose always to see the couple together and to disclose all information, including telephone conversations, to both partners. Clinicians should be guided by their theoretical orientation and professional or ethical judgment. When partners cannot be clear or honest with each other, therapy usually becomes confusing and frustrating for the therapist. This might signal to the therapist that the topic of infidelity needs to be explored. It also could be inappropriate to work on the couple's relationship if the affair is continuing. A therapeutic separation (discussed later in this chapter) may be a reasonable response. Individual work with a partner who is ambivalent about both marital and extramarital relationships can be done before a commitment to couple work is made.

If infidelity is identified, a crisis intervention often needs to follow. After this, a clearer definition of the problem can be made to determine if individual or couple therapy should be started. In addition, children may have knowledge or hold emotional secrets for their parents, especially if the infidelity has gone on for some time. This might need to be explored.

Ending the affair is only the first step in this delicate restoration process. It affects both partners, not just the faithful one. The couple is faced with a number of tasks: They must find ways to reestablish trust in the relationship; examine the reasons for the affair, which connects to the dissatisfaction with the relationship; provide time for grief and jealousy to be a part of the relationship for awhile; and find a way to learn from and let go of (forgive) the infidelity in order to commit to a newly defined relationship.

Violence

Both in theory and practice, marital and family therapy has only recently begun to fully address the issue of male violence toward females. Despite the frequency, lethality, and cost of domestic violence, many therapists fail to detect it. Further, the perpetrator's role isn't adequately addressed by a systemic view that focuses on the reciprocal nature of problems. The violent partner (usually a man) must take full responsibility for his behavior and recognize that violence cannot be part of a healthy relationship. An understanding of how societal and gender factors affect this issue must be incorporated into our clinical work with domestic violence. Also, social and cultural norms must be understood and sometimes challenged. Of course, taking this posture makes it more difficult to therapeutically align with the violent partner.

Recently improved domestic violence programs take a community-wide perspective of the problem. The focus today is on enhancing responses of police and the courts, providing psychoeducation that focuses on beliefs and behaviors of perpetrators and victims, and offering couple therapy that examines interpersonal patterns and teaches skills to better manage conflict and anger.

When faced with a domestic violence case, the therapist's first step is to determine if the victim is safe. The couple should be separated if this cannot be assured. The first treatment goal is to eliminate the violence. If the offending partner won't commit to a "no violence" contract or can't take ownership for violent behavior, then it is wise to separate the couple into group or individual treatment before embarking on conjoint therapy.

Therapists need to examine their own beliefs and reactions to domestic violence, especially given its emotional intensity, the potential danger involved, and the effect of any prior victimization of the therapist. Moral, legal, and ethical concerns related to this issue must be well thought out by the therapist in order to respond professionally. Solid supervision must be available when a beginning therapist first encounters this difficult and, sadly, all-too-common aspect of couple work.

Sexual Difficulties

Problems in sexual functioning often comingle with complaints in other couple relationship areas. In a perfect systemic example we see that a couple's fights at the kitchen table impact how they communicate in bed, and how they communicate in bed affects their fights at the kitchen table. Understanding a couple's relational health (or lack of it) requires information on sexual functioning, in addition to other domains.

Some sexual difficulties stem from simple mechanical or behavioral problems, and respond well to brief sex therapy techniques. Brief sex therapy includes sexual conditioning, deconditioning, and other specific tasks assigned to the individual or couple. This approach is particularly helpful for orgasmic dysfunctions and excitement problems. Of course, the therapist needs to know if the partners have undergone medical examinations to rule out or clarify any biological causes. It's also important to check if clients are using any medications that might interfere with sexual functioning.

When sexual problems are a significant focus in the beginning of therapy, a sexual history should be taken. Even if absolutely no mention is made of the couple's sexual relationship, the therapist should still inquire about any sexual difficulties. The onset and context of a sexual complaint should be explored so that contributing factors are clarified. Expectations and ignorance about sexuality can be identified, as can gender and cultural differences. These factors all play a role in the couple's effort to form a "new system"—a system that will function in sexual and other areas of life. Therapists should also assess for substance use, abuse, or addiction that might impair the couple's sexual relationship. Sometimes a more thorough individual sexual history needs to be taken by one partner if it appears his or her background is significantly affecting the current sexual relationship.

Once the therapist has identified the context of the sexual problems, either a focus on briefer sex therapy will be taken or the sexual problems will be incorporated into the broader framework of therapy. For example, from a transgenerational perspective, the couple could look at generational patterns regarding sexuality and how these patterns are currently impacting their sexual relationship. From a strategic perspective, the therapist might explore how the couple's sexual problems tie into the way the couple "makes up" after a fight. From an experiential perspective, a couple's sexual problems tie to unacknowledged anger and resentment that "somaticize" into low sexual desire. From any perspective, sexual difficulties can be addressed appropriately by many of the tools used in couple therapy in general.

Same-Sex Couples

Most of the information written in this chapter applies to any couple. However, several areas need to be addressed that are unique to providing therapy for same-sex couples. First, in gender socialization, same-sex partners have been exposed to essentially the same gender patterns—that is, most same sex couples are well socialized into their own gender roles. The therapist must understand the strengths and deficits of each gender role since these impact how the couple might be having difficulty functioning. For example, intimacy patterns are more sexually prominent in gay relationships and more emotionally prominent in lesbian relationships. Men tend to merge money later in their relationship development than do women. Relationship maintenance for gay men may be more "work" than for lesbian women, since gender-role socialization assists women in the skills required. In contrast, tolerance for separateness might be more available in gay male relationships that in lesbian ones. The therapist working with same-sex couples does well to understand gender identity development and to use this information to help the couple understand the presenting problems.

A second consideration includes the social reactions and cultural limitations faced by same-sex couples. More than half of the states in the United States carry laws that criminalize forms of sexual expression most common to lesbians and gay men. Data from national lesbian and gay rights organizations show many homosexuals have experienced violence related to sexual orientation (Berrill, 1990). Lesbian and gay men cannot usually designate their partners for work-related benefits or health insurance, nor can they be easily recognized as a "legal family" that can visit intensive care patients or make medical decisions. Few models or cultural ceremonies are available for gay or lesbian couples to support their relationships. Families often shun, distance, ignore, or attack couples attempting to identify and honestly express their commitment. Same-sex couples themselves may internalize these negative reactions and attack their own partners using these ideas. Thus, many same-sex couples are isolated from broader family ties and experience ambivalence within their own relationships.

Finally, therapists need to access other support systems in order to address the unique needs of gay and lesbian couples. For example, family therapy can incorporate nonbiologically related individuals into the therapeutic system. Special resources available to those couples facing AIDS and HIV issues need to be accessed since many gay male couples face chronic illness or death within their pairings. Each partner also may go through a developmental sequence related to "coming out." For example, one partner might pressure the other to tell family about the relationship before the partner is ready to do this. This pressure can cause conflict in the relationship, but stems from each partner being at a different developmental place. When the couple is nested in a supportive and understanding social network, then this developmental process can be normalized.

Therapists must determine whether or not they can work with same-sex couples. They must learn the preferred nomenclature of the couple they work with (lesbian, gay) and they must research and access community resources whenever possible. The following case example demonstrates that couple work with same-sex partners, like other family therapy, requires attention to individual, dyadic, intergenerational, and cultural issues.

Susan and Brenda are a lesbian couple, each partner in her 40s. They have been living together for the past 4 years, and were "married" 3 years ago in a private commitment ceremony. Presenting problems include constant arguing, verbal abuse, an inability to problem solve together, and a lack of intimacy. They fight about virtually everything from household responsibilities to money, sex, and how to spend their leisure time. Both report being very dissatisfied with the relationship. The arguments have led to several separations, during which Brenda stayed with her mother. Although neither report any physical abuse, there have been moments of pushing and shoving, and Brenda reports being afraid of Susan.

The arguments can generate a great deal of emotion, including anger, fear, and rage. Susan says that Brenda is not committed enough to the relationship, that she won't engage enough in discussions about the relationship, and that she withdraws from contact and closeness. Brenda feels intimidated, bullied, criticized, and threatened by Susan. She sees Susan as being unhappy with whatever she does, and feels that she's not ever good enough to meet Susan's high expectations. They do report periods in which they get along well and enjoy each other's company, as long as they keep things superficial.

Susan is a bright, well-educated, 45-year-old African American woman. She works full time as an elementary school principal. The job is demanding and she likes it very much. She says that she "gives to others all day long" and wants to be given to at home sometimes. She comes from a family of three children, and is not particularly close to her younger brother and sister. She describes her mother as "good, caring, and warm." She was physically and verbally abused by her father. She says that she "still hates him" and is frightened that when she gets angry she becomes just like him. Susan was married to a man when she was 25; the marriage lasted 5 years. She left that relationship for another woman. That partnership lasted 4 years, and was filled with turmoil.

Brenda is a 43-year-old Caucasian woman who is also bright and college educated. She works part-time as a reference librarian. She is an only child and spends much of her time with her ailing grandmother. She has a history of depression and is being treated with antidepressants. During the couple therapy, her depressive symptoms worsened and she felt so overwhelmed that she wasn't able to function in the relationship. She was referred to individual therapy, which proved quite helpful. Brenda feels insecure in the relationship with Susan. She was involved with another woman at the time she met Susan. She reports having felt pressure from Susan to marry.

Susan and Brenda feel frustrated with each other. There has been a lot of blaming and protection of their own feelings. They are both committed to the relationship but can't handle the conflict. Their families are supportive and accepting of the relationship. Susan is active in the gay and lesbian community and has been "out" since her marriage ended. Brenda is "out" with some friends and family but keeps her sexual preference a secret at work.

Treatment of this couple will need to focus on managing conflict more effectively. Personal and family histories will prove valuable in assisting the couple and the therapist in evaluating their style of conflict and developing some ways to contain and manage it.

STRUCTURED SEPARATION

A structured separation can be used as a "cooling off" period when a couple is involved in intense conflict that isn't currently resolvable. Orderly separations are likely to be less destructive than separations that are disorderly and not anticipated (Ahrons, 1994). Some partners will view any separation as "the end of the marriage" and will have great difficulty with the notion that some structured time apart may be useful. Establishing clear boundaries and negotiating times for contact will be helpful in lowering their anxiety. Expectations regarding visits, telephone contacts, dating, parenting, financial and household responsibilities, and therapy need to be discussed. Specificity in establishing frequency of contacts and who shall initiate the contacts might be necessary.

Nichols (1988) has identified three tasks for the couple involved in a decision to divorce. These same tasks seem appropriate when working with a structured separation:

1. Accepting the reality that a separation/divorce is occurring (regardless of how or by whom the decision is made).
2. Coping with the initial emotional/psychological reactions.
3. Performing the initial planning for the contemplated actions.

The therapist can assist the couple in orchestrating the separation and accomplishing the tasks identified by Nichols.

It is typical for one partner to be asking for a separation while the other desires to stay together and "work things out." A prelude to a prolonged physical separation can be one of the spouses taking a vacation or even structuring time apart. However, if one of the spouses is adamant that he or she insists upon a separation, then the therapist can be a helpful mediator. The therapist must be sensitive to each person's concerns and avoid developing a coalition with one of the partners.

Evaluating the style and severity of conflict is necessary when working with couples who are separating. If the conflict is severe and chaotic, then the couple should have limited contact and possibly be instructed not to try to solve problems outside therapy, at least initially. If they're less conflictual and able to spend time together in a congenial atmosphere without quickly escalating into difficulties, then they might gradually increase the amount of time they spend together. Spouses need to be able to adhere to the rules of the separation agreement and reestablish trust in each other. If boundaries are violated, then that trust becomes difficult to create. Consequently, rules and boundaries should be fair and realistic for both parties.

Counseling couples can be more challenging than counseling individuals. The new therapist must strive toward facilitating the creation of a new system or may be called upon to orchestrate a structured separation. Regardless of the goals of therapy, the therapist must strive to structure a therapeutic triangle as this is the framework in which couple therapy occurs.

9

When a Family Member
Has a Mental Illness

"I'm convinced there is nothing we cannot cure." One of the authors heard this comment from a senior therapist who had just returned from an upbeat training seminar in the late 1970s. At that time, the author was an inexperienced student therapist. Nevertheless, she questioned the possibility of "cure" for the serious and long-standing struggles her clients faced.

Twenty-five years later, we have learned that some mental illnesses are intractable despite our best treatment efforts. Families with a mentally ill member may appear at your office door after years of struggle. The illness may have subsumed the family's resources and the individual's identity. Nevertheless, family therapists have much to offer these overextended families. Regardless of the diagnosis, a number of factors influence families with mentally ill members. Loneliness, lack of social support, and increased stressful life events can make the patient or family's situation worse. Family discord, including frequent hostility, conflict, and overinvolvement can also hurt families. In contrast, a strong sense of family identity, closeness, and shared values and beliefs can strengthen and protect families. While keeping these relational qualities in mind, family therapists must also know about individual assessment and diagnosis when working with families of the mentally ill.

INDIVIDUAL AND FAMILY CONCEPTS

In the last 20 years, significant gains have been made in describing mental disorders and discovering effective treatments. The National Insti-

169

tute of Mental Health (NIMH) has sponsored important research examining mental disorders that affect millions of people. Some of this work has looked at promising new treatments such as cognitive-behavioral therapy for panic disorder or psychoeducational approaches for schizophrenia. New research initiatives are being encouraged in the realm of child and adolescent disorders (Kessler, Eaton, Wittchen, & Zhao, 1994).

A growing body of literature examines research on effective treatments for individual disorders. Cognitive-behavioral treatments, interpersonal treatments, and psychoanalytic treatments have been used in field trials for specific disorders. There is a growing awareness that one treatment might not work for every problem, and a current trend to match specific therapies with certain disorders.

In addition to the research on talk therapies, there is a burgeoning literature on the effectiveness of pharmacological treatments. New medications are coming out almost daily to treat disorders that were once considered untreatable. The introduction of Prozac created a public awareness of psychopharmacological medications, and people began to demand the pills that reputedly could change a personality and transform a life. Current research is looking at the efficacy of a "split treatment model"—a combination of talk therapy and medication.

We now know that mental illness can run in families and that transmission may not result only from dysfunctional family patterns, but also involves biological determinants. More often than not, when one mentions family history in a psychological assessment, it refers to genetic transmission. Individual diagnosticians are very interested in relatives both in the present and past who have a history of mental illness, because this suggests genetic transmission in the patient.

Research on genetic transmission was enlightening news to family members of the mentally ill. After years of subtly being blamed for their family member's problems by concepts such as the "schizophrenogenic mother," families were both saddened and relieved to learn the illness has a genetic component. While these discoveries relieve the family of guilt and responsibility for "causing" their family member's illness, it also can give some discouraging news about prognosis and transmission to future generations.

Families will be interested to know that while they did not cause mental illness in one member, they can influence its course. Research on "expressed emotion" and "communication deviance" in schizophrenic families demonstrates that family qualities like overinvolvement, hostility, and critical attitudes can cause the schizophrenic family member to relapse. More recently, hostility and conflict in the family have been examined in relation to depression, dementia, and a variety of other disorders.

This research has demonstrated the powerful impact family behaviors and mood can have on its members and their illnesses.

Family therapists can consider psychiatric consultation for the individual family member with mental illness. The consultation can provide information that the therapist can integrate into the overall treatment plan. In addition, the psychiatrist might recommend psychotropic medication to treat the symptoms of the individual's mental disorder.

To some extent, family therapy has remained separate from these trends (Shields, Wynne, McDaniel, & Gawuisler, 1994). One explanation is that, until recently, family therapists refused to recognize individual diagnosis. The IP simply was the symptom bearer for the family's dysfunction (Denton, 1990). The early years of family therapy can be characterized as a time of differentiating family therapy from all others, and one of its classic traits was the belief that individual mental disorders did not exist. Instead, the individual and his or her problems were to be viewed only in the context of the family and its interaction. Early training in family therapy emphasized treating the entire family, which meant having everybody present in every session. Some early family therapists would go so far as to cancel the session if the entire family wasn't available.

Another reason family therapy may have remained separate from advances in individual diagnosis is that most of these advances came from empirical research. While early family therapists (such as the Palo Alto group) often considered themselves researchers–clinicians, more recently family therapy has been the domain of clinicians. Many of these clinicians have had a skeptical attitude about the value of empirical research in informing their work. Instead, family therapy has been characterized by charismatic leaders presenting new models of therapy that frequently had little or no empirical testing or support.

Lately, family therapy has been strongly influenced by social constructivism. This branch of philosophy suggests that there is no external reality to be discovered, only the realities that people create. Applying these ideas to therapy has led to an emphasis on subjectivity and treating the patient's story or the story co-created by patient and therapist as "reality."

Family therapists strongly influenced by social constructivism and narrative approaches would have little use for descriptive criteria of symptoms and syndromes. As a result of an almost isolationist, antiempirical stance, family therapists remained largely uninformed about recent advances in individual diagnosis. In addition, leaders in individual diagnosis research largely ignored family therapy.

Beginning family therapists can glean useful therapeutic tools from the world of individual diagnosis and simultaneously incorporate the strengths of family therapy. Therapists do not need to choose one ideological position to the exclusion of all other perspectives. Beginning family therapists can use multiple sources of information and perspectives to create an optimal treatment plan for their clients.

INDIVIDUAL DIAGNOSIS IN A FAMILY CONTEXT

Recent epidemiological research suggests that more than 50% of the population will have a mental disorder at some time in their lives. While this statistic may refer to a problem as simple as an "adjustment disorder," the frequency of mental health problems suggests the need for effective treatments. While most people who have a mental health problem improve spontaneously and without treatment, there is a small minority, approximately 14%, who have recurring episodes of mental illness, often at least three major episodes during their lifetime. In addition to this statistic, researchers and clinicians also note that one patient frequently has several problems (comorbidity). Epidemiological data and clinical experience suggest that mental problems of various durations and intensities are frequent, debilitating, and painful for both the person and his or her family (Kessler et al., 1994).

People often have mental health problems that do not meet DSM-IV diagnostic criteria or are not multiple in nature. For the individual diagnostician who closely follows DSM-IV diagnostic outlines, the risk exists that serious problems which do not fit neatly into a category can be overlooked. This poses a more serious risk for children and adolescents because their problems fit DSM-IV criteria less frequently than adult disorders, and can be strongly influenced by developmental issues, which might be overlooked by the diagnostician completing a symptom checklist. A contextual, holistic, constructivist approach to mental health problems can correct for many of these weaknesses.

The most common DSM-IV disorders are mood disorders (such as depression), anxiety disorders, and substance abuse problems. Frequently, a patient suffers from two or more of these disorders simultaneously. While everyone suffers from depression or anxiety at some time in their lives, illness does not refer to these everyday problems but to known, recognizable syndromes. Specificity of symptoms, duration, and intensity distinguish a syndrome from the common problems of living.

However, clinicians and patients often find the distinction between a syndrome and everyday problems unilluminating. A patient who is going through a divorce, working as a single parent, and worried about losing her job doesn't care whether she meets four or five criteria for major depression to justify this diagnosis. She just wants to feel better and her therapist wants to help her. In addition, patients with non-DSM-IV problems such as chronic pain, marital problems, or physical illness simply want relief, not a diagnosis.

As a result, clinicians primarily utilize DSM-IV when it comes to filling out forms or for reimbursement purposes. However, when doing treatment, they focus on the most comprehensive view of the problem(s) that often expands beyond a DSM-IV diagnosis. While the vast majority of family therapists are trained in individual diagnosis (Denton et al., 1997), they may initially disregard individual symptom assessment in order to obtain a more holistic understanding of the patient and his or her family's problems, and to briefly enter the patient's world with as few distractions as possible.

The practical, ethical, and logistical dilemmas of using both individual and family diagnosis have never been clearly delineated. Family therapists have discussed some of the inherent strengths and weaknesses of combining individual and family approaches in assessment and treatment (Clarkin et al., 1988). For the most part, the family therapist has been left the task of working out the nuances of integrating individual and family approaches.

How can a family therapist effectively integrate information on individual diagnosis and still maintain a systemic, contextual, holistic perspective? Perhaps this is possible by maintaining an attitude of openness—a willingness to consider the possibility of individual diagnosis, while still maintaining the strengths of a family therapy approach.

Research on health and illness suggests that loneliness and lack of social support is one of the strongest predictors of decline and further suffering, regardless of the problem. Loss of an important relationship through death, divorce, or other means is rated as one of the most significant stressors a person can experience. Family therapy's strength is its recognition of the importance of these relationships, regardless of the other mental health problems an individual experiences. Being isolated and having no social support can signal problems.

Research on manic–depressive illness and other affective disorders suggests that while individual symptoms can be recognized and perhaps treated with medication or by other means, the symptomatic person still desires the support and love of family (Clarkin & Glick, 1992). In addition, the individual can be either hurt or helped by familial responses. A family therapist can successfully combine in his or her work the basic tenets of systemic thinking with careful attention to individual problems and the clinical literature on both systemic and individual perspectives.

Clearly, the therapist must pay attention to the symptoms of the IP as well as to the characteristics and symptoms of other family members. Questions to think about include the following: "Does this person have a known, recognizable cluster of symptoms that meet specific diagnostic criteria? Should this individual receive treatment for these symptoms, in addition to any other therapeutic goals? Do I, as the therapist, have the skills and knowledge to recognize and treat this problem, or should I consider referral to someone else?"

While most family therapists can recognize symptoms of common problems such as depression or anxiety, they may not spot less frequently occurring syndromes. For example, family therapy students may be unfamiliar with signs indicating Tourette's syndrome or trichotillomania. There are several remedies for this situation.

First, family therapists should make every effort to keep up with the literature on individual diagnosis. In addition, family therapists can maintain an attitude of curiosity and alertness to clinical situations they haven't encountered in the past. Frequent reflection on one's clinical case load and increased supervision for beginning therapists invites further exploration of clinically unfamiliar situations. When the unusual happens, the therapist can begin by consulting colleagues and reading.

Referral to a psychotherapist with expertise in a specific diagnosis is always an option. For example, many family therapists will not treat a family whose adolescent has an eating disorder unless they have significant previous experience in that area. They recognize the severity of the condition and, while they may continue family therapy for other issues or related problems, they make sure the adolescent gets an appropriate referral to a psychotherapist or physician who knows how to treat eating disorders.

Finally, family therapists need to be aware of individual diagnosis because the emerging health care system demands it. As more therapists are paid by health maintenance organizations or other large payer organizations, they will be expected to diagnose and plan treatment according to commonly known protocol. Even when family therapy is a common and highly regarded treatment, familiarity with individual diagnosis will be essential to obtain treatment authorization and fulfill insurance form requirements.

While it would be impossible to describe every individual problem and its treatment here, the rest of this chapter will focus on three of the most common individual disorders: depression, anxiety, and substance abuse. At times, these problems are described as discrete entities, but family therapists recognize that even these disorders are best viewed in a holistic context. A contextual approach makes room for consideration of primary symptoms, other social and emotional problems, and the family's extant strengths and deficits.

DEPRESSION

When individual diagnosticians talk about mood disorders, they refer to specific criteria or symptoms—something beyond the "blues" that everyone experiences at one time or another. The most common syndromes include bipolar disorder, cyclothymia, dysthymia, and major depression. Depressive symptoms appear in other disorders, such as atypical depression, adjustment disorder with depressed mood, and schizoaffective disorder, but these many and varied descriptions are beyond the scope of this book. For family therapists, it is important to note that child and adolescent depression have different pathways and presentation than depression in adults. For example, depression in children frequently presents with irritability.

The prevalence of depression in the general population is high and on the rise (U.S. Department of Health and Human Services, 1993). Up to one in eight individuals may require treatment for depression in their lifetime. However, the majority of depressed people never receive any treatment, if they do, it is usually from their primary care physician, not their family therapist.

Besides being painful, depression can be debilitating and recurring. Bipolar depression is characterized by swings between elated moods (manic episodes) and depressed moods, while cyclothymia is characterized by a more mild manifestation of the same swings. Dysthymia refers to a type of depression that has lasted for at least 2 years and whose symptoms are less debilitating than major depression. Major depression, meanwhile, is a condition in which intense feelings of sadness, loss, and helplessness prevail, to the point of impairing daily functioning. Table 9.1 provides a quick reference of major mood disorders, as well as diagnostic criteria for two components: a major depressive episode, and a manic episode.

Depression occurs twice as often in women as in men (McGrath, Keita, Strickland, & Russon, 1990). Possible explanations include women's characteristic style of internalizing problems (thinking instead of doing) compared to men's more aggressive and externalizing style. The social circumstances of women (living in poverty, or suffering abuse) also play a role. Many mental health experts consider depression in women almost epidemic.

Major risk factors for depression include a family history of depression (regardless of whether this is due to interactional or biological factors), lack of social support, stressful life events, and suicides by family members. In addition, depression frequently is found in individuals who suffer from anxiety or have substance abuse problems. While most patients recover from depression without treatment, they are at high risk for relapse. In addition, the most rigorous study ever completed on treatment for depression found that only 19–32% of recovered patients stayed well for more than a year (Shea, Gibbons, Elkin, & Sotsky, 1995).

The symptoms of bipolar illness (manic–depressive disorder) are often dramatic and intense, and the majority of bipolar patients will experience about 11 episodes of either mania (elated mood) or depression (sad, tear-

TABLE 9.1. Quick Reference for Mood Disorders

Disorder	Description
Major depressive disorder	Characterized by one or more major depressive episode (e.g., at least 2 weeks of depressed mood or loss of interest accompanied by at least four additional symptoms of depression).
Dysthymic disorder	Characterized by at least 2 years of depressed mood for more days than not, accompanied by additional depressive symptoms that do not meet criteria for a major depressive episode.
Bipolar I disorder	Characterized by one or more manic or mixed episodes, usually accompanied by major depressive episodes.
Bipolar II disorder	Characterized by one or more major depressive episodes accompanied by at least one hypomanic episode.
Cyclothymic disorder	Characterized by at least 2 years of numerous periods of hypomanic symptoms that do not meet criteria for a manic episode and numerous periods of depressive symptoms that do not meet criteria for a major depressive episode.

Criteria for major depressive episode[a]

A. Five (or more) of the following symptoms have been present during the same 2-week period and represent a change from previous functioning; at least one of the symptoms is either (1) depressed mood or (2) loss of interest of pleasure . . .

(1) depressed mood most of the day, nearly every day, as indicated by either subjective report (e.g., feels sad or empty) or observation made by others (e.g., appears tearful). **Note:** In children and adolescents, can be irritable mood.

(2) markedly diminished interest or pleasure in all, or almost all, activities most of the day, nearly every day (as indicated by either subjective account or observation made by others)

(3) significant weight loss when not dieting or weight gain (e.g., a change of more than 5% of body weight in a month), or decrease or increase in appetite nearly every day. **Note:** In children, consider failure to make expected weight gains.

(4) insomnia or hypersomnia nearly every day

(5) psychomotor agitation or retardation nearly every day (observable by others, not merely subjective feelings of restlessness or being slowed down)

(6) fatigue or loss of energy nearly every day

(7) feelings of worthlessness or excessive or inappropriate guilt (which may be delusional) nearly every day (not merely self-reproach or guilt about being sick)

(8) diminished ability to think or concentrate, or indecisiveness, nearly every day (either by subjective account or as observed by others)

(9) recurrent thoughts of death (not just fear of dying), recurrent suicidal ideation without a specific plan, or a suicide attempt or a specific plan for committing suicide

(cont.)

TABLE 9.1. (cont.)

B. The symptoms do not meet criteria for a mixed episode.

C. The symptoms cause clinically significant distress or impairment in social, occupational, or other important areas of functioning.

D. The symptoms are not due to the direct physiological effects of a substance (e.g., a drug of abuse, a medication) or a general medical condition (e.g., hypothyroidism).

E. The symptoms are not better accounted for by bereavement i.e., after the loss of a loved one, the symptoms persist for longer than 2 months or are characterized by marked functional impairment, morbid preoccupation with worthlessness, suicidal ideation, psychotic symptoms, or psychomotor retardation.

Criteria for manic episode[b]

A. A distinct period of abnormally and persistently elevated, expansive, or irritable mood, lasting at least 1 week (or any duration if hospitalization is necessary.)

B. During the period of mood disturbance, three (or more) of the following symptoms have persisted (four if the mood is only irritable) and have been present to a significant degree:

(1) inflated self-esteem or grandiosity
(2) decreased need for sleep (e.g., feels rested after only 3 hours of sleep)
(3) more talkative than usual or pressure to keep talking
(4) flight of ideas or subjective experience that thoughts are racing
(5) distractibility (i.e., attention too easily drawn to unimportant or irrelevant external stimuli)
(6) increase in goal-directed activity (either socially, at work or school, or sexually) or psychomotor agitation
(7) excessive involvement in pleasurable activities that have a high potential for painful consequences (e.g., engaging in unrestrained buying sprees, sexual indiscretions, or foolish business investments)

C. The symptoms do not meet criteria for a mixed episode.

D. The mood disturbance is sufficiently severe to caused marked impairment in occupational functioning or in usual social activities or relationships with others, or to necessitate hospitalization to prevent harm to self or others, or there are psychotic features.

E. The symptoms are not due to the direct physiological effects of a substance (e.g., a drug of abuse, a medication, or other treatment) or a general medical condition (e.g., hyperthyroidism).

[a]From American Psychiatric Association (1994, p. 327). Copyright 1994 by the American Psychiatric Association. Reprinted by permission.

[b]From American Psychiatric Association (1994, p. 332). Copyright 1994 by the American Psychiatric Association. Reprinted by permission.

ful, hopeless mood) during their lifetime (Davenport & Adland, 1988). In addition, manic–depressive illness is seldom "cured," but managed throughout a person's life. A family who witnesses an initial episode in one of its members can expect more of the same in years to come. These bouts can leave a family reeling and wondering when the next "crazy" episode will happen (Pittman, 1987). One family powerfully described their confusion when police told them that their college son threw a microwave oven through a store window. Their story chronicles years of treatment, confusion, feeling blamed, and eventual healing after their son and brother was diagnosed with manic–depressive illness (Berger & Berger, 1991).

Recently, family therapy has been examined as a treatment for major depression and dysthymia, and work at Cornell University has looked at using couple group therapy in cases where one member of the dyad has bipolar disorder (Clarkin & Glick, 1992; Moltz, 1993). A close relationship with a depressed person is difficult at best. The relationship can be challenged by the sad, hopeless quality the depressed person emanates or the dramatic swings in mood and behavior of the bipolar patient. In addition, the depressed person may look to significant others to help them cope or, even worse, they may withdraw from relationships completely.

The family's response to the depressed person can be a key influence in the course of the depression (Clarkin et al., 1988). Some of the most impressive work on depression (Bergin & Garfield, 1994) has examined marital therapy, especially behavioral marital therapy, as a form of treatment. Results of these outcome studies demonstrate that for women who received marital therapy to treat depression, the marriage improved and the depression abated. This is in contrast to women who received individual treatment, in which only the depressive symptoms abated. Treating depression with marital therapy makes sense, especially when one considers that the most prevalent patient is a wife or mother, in her late 20s to early 40s, who is socially isolated and depressed about her relationship with her husband. If the marriage is not distressed, individual therapy may be equally useful (Alexander, Holtzworth-Munroe, & Jameson, 1994).

In discussing social and family relationships of depressed persons, Gotlib and Beach (1995) state:

> Whereas depressed persons exhibit social skills deficits in their interactions with strangers, their interactions with their spouse and children are more likely to be characterized by hostility and anger . . . it is clear that depression in one family member has a significant influence on the emotions and behavior of other members and . . . on the family as a unit. Conversely, negative interactions with spouse or other family members are powerfully related to level of depressive symptomatology. (p. 418)

While no research suggests that families cause depression in individuals, studies indicate that family members affect the course of the illness (Keitner, Ryan, Miller, & Kohn, 1993; Sprenkle & Bischoff, 1991). Many researchers suggest a reciprocal relationship between depression and family interaction, stating that it is impossible to identify a single etiology. Yet Clarkin et al. (1988) suggest that "emotional support from an intimate partner, and the perception that one has access to a range of support if needed . . . insulate against life stress and decrease the risk for depression" (p. 15).

On the negative side, criticism and continued hostility seem to have an onerous effect on both the depressed person and the family. In one study, the strongest predictor of posthospital symptom course was a depressed woman's perception of the support she received from her spouse (Goering & Rhodes, 1994). The same study noted that women who were married more than 7 years and had unsupportive marriages were the least likely to recover. The author suggests that the depressed woman's perception of her marital support may be a better prognostic indicator than the clinical characteristics of the depressive illness. In addition, some research suggests that depressed patients tend to relapse at lower levels of criticism than do schizophrenic patients (Keitner et al., 1993). Clearly, family support (especially spousal support) is critical in the course and treatment of depression (Miklowitz & Goldstein, 1997).

Some research suggests that spouses of depressed persons may be empathic to their partner's suffering at first, but over time become impatient and even hostile (Clarkin et al., 1988). The therapist and family confront a challenging situation when the hostile spouse identifies the reason for that hostility as the partner's "helpless behavior" and the depressed spouse claims a need for the partner's "love and support" to improve.

The influence of criticism, contempt, defensiveness, and withdrawal in couples with a depressed partner are important because these same themes predict marital deterioration and divorce (Gottman, 1994). In addition, distress and psychopathology in parents predict the same in children. Depression is not an isolated illness residing within an individual, but a serious condition that affects every family relationship, and even the continuing existence of the family.

Clarkin and Glick (1992) point out the change in attitudes of professionals toward depressed patients and their families by noting mental health workers' growing recognition of the burden of mental illness. Instead of blaming the family (or spouse) for causing the illness, professionals need to empathize with the challenge inherent in daily life with a depressed member. Common issues family members may present with include the degree of responsibility one must assume for the depressed member, suppressing or denying one's own feelings or needs, globalizing the illness and blaming all negative behaviors and family interactions on the illness, and arguing with the spouse about treatment recommendations such as medication compliance and therapy.

A family therapist's ability to provide support, education, and information about depression can affect not only the individual patient but the marital and parenting relationships as well. Family therapists can assess not only for the individual symptoms of depression but for the impact the depressed person's mood and behaviors have on other family members and the group's overall well-being. Spouses and children of depressed parents can be considered an integral part of the treatment.

In particular, the intertwined relationship between an individual's depression (especially a woman's), the marriage, and parenting need careful examination. Treatment should be multifaceted, addressing each of these issues and their overlap. Perhaps in no other mental disorder has such a clear relationship been demonstrated than that between marital quality and the course of the disorder. In addition, children's therapists lament that adult therapists often overlook the impact of parental problems on children's development. Family therapists treating depressed parents have the opportunity to assess and treat the children who are affected by their parent's emotional states.

A summary of outcome studies looking at a marital format to treat depression suggests that women with unipolar depression who are distressed about their marriage can be effectively treated with marital therapy (Prince & Jacobson, 1995). The patient's perception of the problem is important in deciding what type of treatment to pursue. The therapist can assess how central the marital relationship is in the patient's beliefs about why she is depressed.

Less work has been done looking at family therapy to treat depression, but evidence suggests that parent–child disputes are prominent in families with a depressed member (Gotlib & Beach, 1995). In addition, evidence exists that depressed children grow up in homes with one or more depressed parents. Thus, family therapy can potentially ameliorate a damaging situation for multiple family members. Family therapies cannot only remediate individual symptomatology of the depressed person, but can potentially improve the marriage and the parent–child relationships.

Current research and information about depression give beginning family therapists several guidelines to follow when working with depressed people and their families:

- Check for a family history of depression.
- Consider medication for the depressed family member as an efficient, cost-effective treatment option.
- Consider how the marital relationship influences the member's depression (by asking him or her).

- Note other family members' responses to the depressed member (e.g., distancing, empathizing, hostility, overinvolvement, criticism)
- When a parent is depressed, assess the impact on the children.
- Look for depression masked as other symptoms (e.g., irritability, anger, withdrawal)
- Consider treatment options including individual therapy (especially cognitive-behavioral treatments), couple therapy, family therapy, and group therapy and match treatment to the specific needs and wishes of the clients.
- Use psychoeducation to inform family members about depression.

Marital and family therapies to treat depression generally work best for clients with mild depression and have been shown to be less effective for those who were part of an inpatient sample of severely depressed persons (Clarkin et al., 1988; Prince & Jacobson, 1995). Marital and family therapies may be used in conjunction with other treatments, such as pharmacotherapy and/ or individual therapy. Psychoeducational and supportive family approaches can be effective for treating bipolar clients and their families.

ANXIETY

Everyone gets anxious and nervous at times—it's the human condition. But true anxiety disorders are more intense and specific than the general worry we all experience. Fortunately, treatments for these disorders have some of the most successful outcome records. In fact, a group of mental health researchers identified cognitive-behavioral treatments for panic disorders as having the most empirical support and success of any matched disorder/treatment in the last 10 years (U.S. Department of Health and Human Services, 1993). New work is going on daily in discovering better pharmacological and cognitive-behavioral treatments for anxiety disorders. While most mental health problems have a 50–70% treatment success rate, some of the anxiety disorders have 70–90% cure rate, particularly panic attack with agoraphobia. With these statistics in mind, a family therapist might consider referral to an individual therapist with expertise in pharmacology or cognitive-behavioral treatments for the individual, while simultaneously continuing to treat the family.

Not all anxiety disorders can be treated effectively, however. For example, posttraumatic stress disorder often is difficult to "cure," but can be managed. Nevertheless, compared to many disorders where the goal is symptom management, one can at times talk about "cure" for some anxiety disorders. Major subtypes of anxiety disorders, as well as diagnostic criteria for two of these (panic attack and generalized anxiety disorder) are highlighted in Table 9.2.

TABLE 9.2. Quick Reference for Anxiety Disorders

Disorder	Description
Panic attack	A discrete period in which there is the sudden onset of intense apprehension, fearfulness, or terror, often associated with feelings of impending doom. See criteria for panic attack for specific symptoms.
Agoraphobia	Anxiety about, or avoidance of, places or situations from which escape might be difficult or embarrassing or in which help may not be available in the event of having a panic attack or panic-like symptoms.
Panic disorder	Without agoraphobia, is characterized by recurrent unexpected panic attacks about which there is persistent concern. With agoraphobia, is characterized by both recurrent unexpected panic attacks and agoraphobia. Without a history of panic disorder, is characterized by agoraphobia and panic-like symptoms.
Specific phobia	Is characterized by clinically significant anxiety provoked by exposure to a specific feared object or situation, often leading to avoidance behavior.
Social phobia	Is characterized by clinically significant anxiety provoked by exposure to certain types of social or performance situations, often leading to avoidance behavior.
Obsessive–compulsive disorder	Is characterized by obsessions (which cause marked anxiety or distress) and/or by compulsions (which serve to neutralize anxiety).
Posttraumatic stress disorder	Is characterized by the reexperiencing of an extremely traumatic event accompanied by symptoms of increased arousal and by avoidance of stimuli associated with the trauma.
Acute stress disorder	Is characterized by symptoms similar to those of posttraumatic stress disorder that occur immediately in the aftermath of an extremely traumatic event.
Generalized anxiety disorder	Is characterized by at least 6 months of persistent and excessive anxiety and worry.

Criteria for panic attack[a]

A discrete period of intense fear or discomfort, in which four (or more) of the following symptoms developed abruptly and reached a peak within 10 minutes:

(1) palpitations, pounding heart, or accelerated heart rate
(2) sweating
(3) trembling or shaking

(cont.)

TABLE 9.2. (cont.)

(4) sensations of shortness of breath or smothering
(5) feeling of choking
(6) chest pain or discomfort
(7) nausea or abdominal distress
(8) feeling dizzy, unsteady, lightheaded, or faint
(9) derealization (feelings of unreality) or depersonalization (being (detached from oneself)
(10) fear of losing control or going crazy
(11) fear of dying
(12) paresthesias (numbness or tingling sensations)
(13) chills or hot flushes

Criteria for generalized anxiety disorder[b]

A. Excessive anxiety and worry (apprehensive expectation), occurring more days than not for at least 6 months, about a number of events or activities (such as work or school performance).

B. The person finds it difficult to control the worry.

C. The anxiety and worry are associated with three (or more) of the following six symptoms (with at least some symptoms present for more days than not for the past 6 months). **Note:** Only one item is required in children.

(1) restlessness or feeling keyed up or on edge
(2) being easily fatigued
(3) difficulty concentrating or mind going blank
(4) irritability
(5) muscle tension
(6) sleep disturbance (difficulty falling or staying asleep, or restless, unsatisfying sleep)

D. The focus of the anxiety and worry is not confined to features of an Axis I disorder, e.g., the anxiety or worry is not about having a panic attack (as in panic disorder), being embarrassed in public (as in social phobia), being contaminated (as in obsessive–compulsive disorder), being away from home or close relatives (as in separation anxiety disorder), gaining weight (as in anorexia nervosa), having multiple physical complaints (as in somatization disorder), or having a serious illness (as in hypochondriasis), and the anxiety and worry do not occur exclusively during posttraumatic stress disorder.

E. The anxiety, worry, or physical symptoms cause clinically significant distress or impairment in social, occupational, or other important areas of functioning.

F. The disturbance is not due to the direct physiological effects of a substance (e.g., a drug of abuse, a medication) or a general medical condition (e.g., hyperthyroidism) and does not occur exclusively during a mood disorder, a psychotic disorder, or a pervasive developmental disorder.

[a]From American Psychiatric Association (1994, p. 395). Copyright 1994 by the American Psychiatric Association. Reprinted by permission.

[b]From American Psychiatric Association (1994, pp. 435–436). Copyright 1994 by the American Psychiatric Association. Reprinted by permission.

Frequently, people suffer from both an anxiety disorder and another major problem: depression or substance abuse. At times, a client may suffer from all three, using the substance to deal with the other two problems. Physicians who prescribe medication often try to delineate the symptoms of each one, and prescribe medication to treat specific symptoms. They also try to understand which cluster of symptoms is dominant. Thus the patient's "primary diagnosis" might be generalized anxiety disorder with symptoms of depression.

These distinctions, while important, may be less critical to a family therapist. While the therapist can profit from identifying specific symptoms of each disorder, the client is treated as a whole person, and symptoms are seen as part of a whole life, not discrete entities. The patient's perspective and family context are equally important.

Anxiety disorders are common, and occur almost twice as often in women than in men. Prevalence of anxiety disorders does not vary, however, on the basis of race, income, education, or rural versus urban living. Once again, we note that women tend to internalize (and become anxious) while men are more likely to externalize or act (perhaps get drunk or become violent) when they are distressed.

Anxiety disorders are the most frequently diagnosed problem of children and adolescents, and some research suggests that anxious children become anxious adults (Dadds, 1995). Children's worries are different from adults', and they have different kinds of fears. They may not want to go to school (as in school phobia), they may be afraid of strangers, or they may not want to leave mother and father (as in separation anxiety). Regardless of the age-appropriate symptoms, anxiety in childhood can be a frightening and debilitating problem.

Since anxiety disorders generally involve how or what an individual is thinking and his or her physiological responses to these thoughts, it's easy to understand why anxiety disorders might be thought of as problems of the individual. Indeed, sometimes anxiety disorders can be effectively and efficiently treated with individual therapies. Pharmacological treatments and cognitive-behavioral treatments are effective for people suffering from anxiety, and have little or no focus on the patient's family.

Cognitive-behavioral treatments focus on changing how people think and behave. An underlying assumption is that if a person changes thinking or behavior, physiology and emotions will change, too. Gradually exposing someone to the situation they most fear and giving them new ways of thinking about it have proven especially useful treatments.

These methods are similar to the structural family therapy techniques of reframing and enactment. In addition, solution-focused therapists suggest "making one small change" in the way one normally behaves about a problem. Narrative therapists talk about someone's "inner dialogue" and "re-storying" one's life. These family therapy approaches share many similarities with cognitive behavioral techniques.

However, clinical literature or research on family approaches to treating anxiety disorders is rare. The existing literature focuses on treating agoraphobia and panic disorder (Craske & Zoellner, 1995). In reviewing the literature on an interpersonal context for panic disorder and agoraphobia, Barlow states, "A review of the literature leads to the conclusion that the concept of a distinct marital system that predisposes to the development of agoraphobia is almost devoid of empirical support . . . [but] marital dissatisfaction may represent one of several possible stressors that precipitates panic attacks" (Barlow, 1993, p. 72).

Craske and Zoellner (1995) summarize the evidence examining the relationship between marital relations and anxiety: "There is evidence . . . that poor marital relations can predict poorer phobia outcome, that certain types of phobia treatment may have detrimental effects upon marital relations, and that marital distress may contribute to the maintenance . . . of panic and agoraphobia" (p. 398).

Barlow also suggests that marital distress has been found to adversely affect responses to cognitive–behavioral treatments, and that involvement of the spouse in every aspect of treatment has been found to override the negative impact of poor marital relations on phobic treatment. In other words, the studies suggest the value of including the spouse in treatment for agoraphobia (Barlow, 1993).

Barlow states that negative effects can result if cognitive-behavioral treatments are conducted without the spouse's involvement because major role changes may occur that are beyond the "healthy" partner's perceived control. Simply put, a change in one part of the system (the agoraphobic symptoms of the spouse) affects all parts of the system.

As stated earlier, the major focus for marital therapy in anxiety disorders is agoraphobia and panic. New research is just beginning to incorporate spouses in the treatment of obsessive-compulsive disorder, social phobia, generalized anxiety disorder, and posttraumatic stress disorder. Existing evidence on outcomes for these disorders suggests that social support—especially family support—leads to superior outcomes. Negative family interactions such as criticism, anger, hostile confrontation, and a spouse's belief that the client could control his or her own symptoms if he or she wished were all predictors of poor outcome (Craske & Zoellner, 1995).

The role of family therapy may be even stronger when treating children with anxiety disorders. Dadds (1995) suggests that fearful, apprehensive responses instead of feelings of mastery and competence are learned by children—often by watching their parents. Some research suggests that anxious children grow up in homes with at least one anxious parent. While the family therapist needs to be careful not to fall into the historical trap of blaming the parents for the origins of the child's problems, he or she needs to understand how each parent responds to anxiety-producing stimuli and what the family's response to fearful situations has been in the past. Family treatments, especially those employing cognitive-behavioral principles, can be effective treatments since family members share many beliefs, including a worldview. In addition, the powerful influence of emotional support from spouses and parents can be directed toward recognizing and praising mastery and competence instead of reinforcing worry.

Family therapists are aware of covert and overt rules and beliefs in the family as well as hidden agendas. Beliefs and hidden agendas strongly influence a person's response to anxiety. For example, a lonely parent may be as ambivalent about a child's going to school as is the youngster. The parent then subtly reinforces "school refusal" behavior. A spouse who is easily threatened and needs to control the lives of his or her family may be content to do all the work for an agoraphobic spouse. Recognizing that change in one part of the family brings change for each member, the family therapist can assess for individual responses as well as the interaction between family members regarding the IP's anxiety.

Many of the guidelines used for treating depression also hold true for treating anxious clients and their families. In addition, current research and information about anxiety disorders provide several clinical guidelines for working with anxious clients and their families:

- For panic disorders and phobias, consider cognitive-behavioral treatments.
- Consider the role family conflict or marital conflict have in influencing the member's anxious symptoms.
- Consider covert or hidden relational interactions that influence the member's anxious symptoms (e.g., the partner's need to "control" and "protect" the anxious member).
- Consider the "place" or "function" of the anxious symptoms in the family system and the marital system.
- When treating anxious children, evaluate how the parents cope with stress and what coping skills they have taught their children.

ALCOHOLISM AND DRUG ABUSE

Substance abuse, whether it involves alcohol, illegal drugs, or prescribed medication, can occur when the therapist least expects it. Unless the therapist works at a drug and alcohol treatment center, few couples or families identify substance abuse as the presenting problem—exactly the opposite usually occurs. The family presents because a child is acting out in school and the school has required therapy for behavior problems. A couple requests marital therapy after years of tension and the wife's recent ultimatum, and the therapist begins treatment only to discover a substance abuse problem.

Individual therapists can simply ask the patient about substance use, but a family therapist may have to search for the abuse before it becomes apparent. The family may be so used to the abuser's behavior that it no longer considers it a problem, at least overtly. Family members may be frightened, ashamed, or intimidated into denying (at least verbally to an "outsider") that there is a substance abuse problem. They can only get to therapy by requesting help for something else. The most important advice for a beginning family therapist is this: Consider the possibility of a substance abuse problem during your assessment, regardless of the presenting problems, and reconsider the possibility every time a constellation of symptoms, explanations, or descriptions do not make sense. Table 9.3 provides a quick reference of DSM-IV diagnostic criteria for substance dependence and abuse.

The professional debates surrounding substance abuse can be confusing to a new therapist who is trying to learn the basics. Current controversies surround the issues of whether an alcoholic can ever drink again, whether alcoholism is a biological disease, whether recreational drug use leads to abuse and addiction, whether an "addictive personality" exists, and whether this personality develops from childhood trauma. Diagnosis is further confused by the arbitrary distinctions made about use, abuse, and dependence.

The beginning family therapist might look at these ongoing controversies as intellectually interesting. However, the therapist developing basic clinical skills also can find these arguments distracting from the primary goal—to get the person to stop using or abusing the substance. One therapist explained the goal of substance abuse work by comparing it to surgery: "I simply want to cut the harmful substance out of the person's life and then I'll do a pathology summary later, when the person is no longer being harmed." Substance abusers, family members, and other professionals can get caught up in myriad debates surrounding substance abuse and never focus on the simple behavioral issue of stopping the problem.

Substance abuse is much more common in men than women. As a result, behaviors that reflect lapses in judgment and reasoning and lack of behavioral control, such as violence and sexual abuse, are much more common in men. If a family therapist scratches the surface of many deviant social behaviors committed by men, he or she will usually find comorbid substance abuse.

TABLE 9.3. Quick Reference for Substance Dependence and Substance Abuse

Criteria for substance dependence[a]

A maladaptive pattern of substance use, leading to clinically significant impairment or distress, as manifested by three (or more) of the following, occurring at any time in the same 12-month period:

(1) tolerance, as defined by either of the following:
    (a) a need for markedly increased amounts of the substance to achieve intoxication or desired effect
    (b) markedly diminished effect with continued use of the same amount of the substance
(2) withdrawal, as manifested by either of the following:
    (a) the characteristic withdrawal syndrome for the substance (refer to [DSM-IV] criteria sets for Withdrawal from specific substances)
    (b) the same (or a closely related) substance is taken to relieve or avoid withdrawal symptoms
(3) the substance is often taken in larger amounts or over a longer period than was intended
(4) there is a persistent desire or unsuccessful efforts to cut down or control substance use
(5) a great deal of time is spend in activities necessary to obtain the substance (e.g., visiting multiple doctors or driving long distances), use the substance (e.g., chain-smoking), or recover from its effects
(6) important social, occupational, or recreational activities are given up or reduced because of substance use
(7) the substance use is continued despite knowledge of having a persistent or recurrent physical or psychological problem that is likely to have been caused or exacerbated by the substance (e.g., current cocaine use despite recognition of cocaine-induced depression, or continued drinking despite recognition that an ulcer was made worse by alcohol consumption.

Criteria for substance abuse[b]

A. A maladaptive pattern of substance use leading to clinically significant impairment or distress, as manifested by one (or more) of the following, occurring within a 12–month period:

    (1) recurrent substance use resulting in a failure to fulfill major role obligations at work, school, or home (e.g., repeated absences or poor work performance related to substance use; substance-related absences, suspensions, or expulsions from school; neglect of children or household)
    (2) recurrent substance use in situations in which it is physically hazardous (e.g., driving an automobile or operating a machine when impaired by substance use)
    (3) recurrent substance-related legal problems (e.g., arrests for substance-related disorderly conduct)
    (4) continued substance use despite having persistent or recurrent social or interpersonal problems caused or exacerbated by the effects of the substance (e.g., arguments with spouse about consequences of intoxication, physical fights)

B. The symptoms have never met the criteria for substance dependence for this class of substance.

[a]See DSM-IV for various specifiers. From American Psychiatric Association (1994, p. 181). Copyright 1994 by the American Psychiatric Association. Reprinted by permission.

[b]From American Psychiatric Association (1994, p. 181–183). Copyright 1994 by the American Psychiatric Association. Reprinted by permission.

Substance abuse is a serious and common problem in the United States, and is related to drunk driving, suicide, homicide, violent crime, child and spouse abuse, and "household accidents." In addition, the biological effects of substance abuse can permanently damage a person's health. Effects include cirrhosis, hepatitis, and seizures. Alcoholism can be a true systemic illness—fetal alcohol syndrome is one of the only illnesses in which the mother does the damaging behavior and the child feels the effects, forever.

Assessment of alcoholism and substance abuse have been addressed in an earlier chapter. The purpose here is to review clinical and research literature that examines the role of alcoholism in the family and effective family treatments. Alcoholism and substance abuse is one of the DSM-IV categories that has received the most investigation by family therapists, perhaps because of evidence that alcoholism and substance abuse are "family diseases" in the sense that the abuser's behavior affects everyone in the family and, in turn, the abuser is affected by family members.

Steinglass's research on alcoholic families suggests that a family's rituals, routines, and beliefs are strongly influenced by alcohol. In essence, the family can take on an "alcoholic identity" and collude to allow the alcoholic behavior to continue. At times, positive effects of the alcohol, not just damaging effects, are experienced by the family. For example, a family may be reluctant to encourage a husband and father who is more relaxed and engaging when he drinks to stop the drinking.

In *The Alcoholic Family,* the authors take a developmental view (Steinglass, Bennett, Wolin, & Reiss, 1987). They suggest the that seeds of an alcoholic family identity are planted early in the marriage, as a couple decides on patterns to follow and beliefs to hold—largely an implicit process. The role of alcohol and drinking in the family, while influenced by family of origin patterns, is one of the "decisions" a new couple makes. In essence, several small "agreements" to accept alcohol and alcoholic behavior can lead to a big "yes," and an alcoholic family is formed.

The authors contend that every alcoholic family must contend with the following characteristics of alcoholism: It is chronic; it involves use of a psychobiologically active drug; it is cyclical in nature; it produces predictable behavioral responses; and it has a definite course of development. Families are more diverse than they are alike in their responses to these issues, and the role of alcohol must be assessed for each individual family.

Recent research reviews and meta-analyses of alcohol and drug studies have examined the efficacy of marital and family treatments for substance abuse, including both alcohol and drugs. McCrady and Epstein (1995) state:

> Research suggests that involving the spouse in treatment increases the probability of a positive outcome in terms of drinking, and that addressing the marital relationship increases the chances of the couple's remaining together and having a more satisfying relationship. (p. 392)

In examining the efficacy of family therapy to treat drug abuse, Liddle and Dakof (1995) state:

> A number of studies from different clinical research groups demonstrate that different versions of family intervention can engage and retain drug users and their families in treatment, significantly reduce drug use and other related problem behaviors, and enhance particular domains of prosocial functioning. Moreover, a smaller number of comparative efficacy studies have shown family therapy to be more effective than non-family therapies. (p. 511)

Edwards and Steinglass (1995) delineate specific situations that influence the efficacy of family treatments for alcoholism. They note that families have a strong influence in motivating alcoholics to get treatment and to alter their drinking behavior. They recommend that family involvement, especially inclusion of nonalcoholic family members in the assessment phase, be a routine component of alcoholism treatment. The impact of family treatment seems to vary according to gender (it is more helpful for men than for women to have spouses involved), investment in the relationship (an investment here produces greater motivation to change drinking behaviors), and support for abstinence from the family.

Most of these studies had control groups and several types of treatment groups, and generally found family therapy to be as effective or more effective than other treatments. Family therapy was almost always superior to no-treatment control groups. Research suggests that involving the nonalcoholic spouse in treatment significantly improves outcome (Jacobson & Gurman, 1995; Steinglass et al., 1987).

Interestingly, many successful drug treatment programs derive from a structural/strategic tradition, while effective alcohol treatment programs derive from a behavioral therapy tradition. Both of these theoretical approaches share an active, problem-solving method with a focus on the present situation. Facilitating communication and problem-solving skills between family members are key elements of these treatments. While there is still much to be learned about treating substance abuse problems or alcoholism with family therapy, one can conclude that an active, focused style is essential for effectiveness.

Beginning clinicians often ask, "Is family therapy or marital therapy enough, or should it be used in conjunction with other forms of treatment?" The answer depends on the specific circumstances of the family. Many family therapy treatments are combined with individual treatments, education programs, and pharmacological treatment. Alexander et al. (1994) comment on using behavioral marital therapy (BMT) as the sole treatment: "Data from studies examining BMT as the sole treatment . . . suggests that this treatment approach leads to less drinking and greater marital satisfaction than other therapeutic approaches" (p. 611).

Some family therapy programs combine aspects of other therapies into the "family approach." For example, Liddle uses an individual therapist to form an alliance with substance abusing adolescents and a separate family therapist to do the family treatment (Liddle & Dakof, 1995). One way to decide whether family therapy should be the sole treatment is to assess the intensity of the family's impact on the problem. For example, family therapy is more effective than other treatments for younger teens but not to the same degree for older teens (Sprenkle & Bischoff, 1991). In addition, behavioral marital therapy or spouse involvement in treatment for alcoholism is more effective for couples who report some marital distress before treatment. The old adage "If it ain't broke, don't fix it" comes to mind. Some research, however, suggests that even couples without marital distress see improved marital satisfaction and communication skills, and prevent deterioration of the relationship, when marital therapy is used to treat substance abuse (Alexander et al., 1994)

In determining whether marital or family therapies should be the sole treatment for a substance problem, the therapist can ask the abuser how much he or she would like the family to participate. On the other hand, limited resources or a structured treatment program may make this decision moot. In general, marital or family therapy should comprise part of the treatment, given the growing evidence of its effectiveness.

Another benefit of including family therapy, besides ameliorating the substance abuse, is improvement in family members' satisfaction with marital and family relationships. When treatment ends, the family has a shared experience and new beliefs to refer back to in times of stress. The spouse can provide reminders of the benefits of the treatment several years after it is over. The potential effects of spouse and family involvement, even when the IP has a substance problem, are noted in the superior follow-up results of family therapy groups compared to other treatment groups.

If the goal is lasting change, not just a quick fix, it makes sense to include the most important people in the abuser's life in treatment because family members will still be with the patient long after therapy has ended. Literature on alcoholism and substance abuse suggest the following clinical guidelines:

- Regardless of presenting problem, consider the possibility and role of substance abuse.

- Assess the role of the alcohol or substance in the family. For example, one family reported that their father was "the most fun and relaxed" when he was drinking, and thus the family saw the drinking as serving some positive functions in the family.
- Consider the possibility of "enabling behaviors" by other family members.
- Assess how pervasive the substance is in influencing family beliefs, rituals, and routines.
- Accept that various family members will have differing views on the seriousness of the substance problem. Some members may minimize the problem and others may focus on the substance use as the key problem in the family.
- Consider the possibility of violence or abuse occurring in the family because they are frequently comorbid with substance use.
- Consider stopping family therapy to treat a different problem and refocusing treatment on stopping the member's substance abuse.

Alcoholism/drug abuse, anxiety, and depression are three of the most common individual disorders a therapist will encounter in a clinical practice. A therapist must not view these disorders in a vacuum but rather within the context of existing and past social and emotional problems and the family's extant strengths and weaknesses. In addition, a therapist must keep in mind that the family of an individual with a mental disorder oftentimes plays an inextricable role in the perpetuation or containment of this disorder and that psychoeducation and support are crucial components to both the family's well-being as well as that of their afflicted family member.

10

Getting Unstuck in Therapy

"I've been working with this family for several weeks, but not much seems to be changing. Now what do I do?" Supervisors and seasoned colleagues often hear this question from beginning therapists. Clearly, therapy is not always a smooth ride for any of its participants, and therapists frequently encounter a multitude of complications and obstacles along the way. Consider the case of the Smith family:

The Smiths initially presented their 16-year-old daughter's sexual acting out as their primary problem. A letter had been discovered by her mother detailing her sexual fantasies and possible encounters with a young man who lived a few hundred miles away. The family sessions included two teenage daughters, ages 16 and 13, and the parents. The family— bright, verbal, and well educated—could express its ideas well, but had considerable difficulty with direct communication and expression of feelings. After several family sessions, the family stabilized and everyone agreed that many of the difficulties were the result of long-standing marital problems.

Couple therapy began as a slow and painful process for the spouses in this family. Considerable sexual tension, a lack of feeling disclosure, and a history of fighting culminated in hurt feelings and emotional withdrawal. The husband had a history of going into rages in which he couldn't control his emotions and would break things in the house. These incidents, described by his wife as "childlike temper tantrums," resulted in the wife withdrawing, becoming depressed, and locking herself in her bedroom. Both individuals harbored a great deal of resentment for past unresolved conflicts dating back to their courtship. The husband insisted that the problem was essentially the wife's. His contention was that her withdrawal and lack of affection caused most of the difficulties. There was no evidence of alcohol abuse. The wife had taken antidepressants on several occasions. These were prescribed by her family doctor—she refused to see a psychiatrist.

The couple therapy progressed for several weeks with little change. The wife refused to talk about her family of origin issues, other than to say she was abused. She indicated that she felt her husband wouldn't understand and would only use the information against her. The husband was willing to discuss his family of origin, but saw little relevancy in it for his marriage. The husband's frustration with the lack of contact and change increased. The wife's depressive symptoms intensified, and included crying spells, sleep problems, withdrawal, excessive worrying, and lethargy. She felt that the marital sessions were "too much" and were creating more stress and difficulty. The husband threatened divorce if his wife didn't change.

Family therapists expect people to be ambivalent about change. The struggle for change is inevitable within any relationship context, including the therapy room. The challenge of facilitating new ways and ending old ways is central to all therapeutic processes. In the following sections, we identify common sources of "stuckness" in therapy and provide options to think about and deal with them.

UNDERSTANDING CLIENTS' AMBIVALENCE ABOUT CHANGE

Beginning therapists need to recognize that a family puts energy and resources into being stuck. Fortunately, the fact that clients even come into therapy usually shows some willingness to try something new or to apply energy in a different way. Further, the therapist's very participation with a client or family can produce and promote change. True change, however, might not be welcomed by the people requesting it. All people have a tendency to go back to the ways things have always been done—homeostasis. Familiar is comfortable.

Resistance is a normal part of therapy, not an exception. Younger therapists sometimes think they have failed when they encounter resistance. In order to talk intelligently about client resistance, we need a definition. For resistance, we use the working definition offered in the excellent text *Mastering Resistance,* by Anderson and Stewart (1983), which states:

> Resistance can be defined as all those behaviors in the therapeutic system which interact to prevent the therapeutic system from achieving the family's goals for therapy. The therapeutic system includes all family members, the therapist, and the context in which the therapy takes place, that is, the agency

or institution in which it occurs. Resistance is most likely to be successful, that is, to result in the termination or failure of family therapy, when resistances are present and interacting synergistically in all three components of the therapeutic system. (p. 24)

Various theoretical orientations label clients' ambivalence about change and their resistance differently. For example, structural family therapy would find resistance in the family's failure to accommodate its structure to the changing developmental needs of its members, while transgenerational family therapies might assess resistance as an integral part of dealing with unfinished business in one's family of origin. Resistance in either case is a predictable partner of change. By definition then, a family therapist must clearly keep in mind both a theoretical approach as well as the family's goals for therapy in order to interpret resistance accurately. Resistance comes with the territory of therapy and must not be viewed as failure, but as an expected aspect of the work.

The client system fears change since it is something new and unpredictable. For example, a client might be an alcoholic, single mother who is coming into therapy because of her child's school problems. If the mother fails to look at the possible influence of her drinking (an examination usually carried out later in the therapeutic relationship) on the child's school problems, we have resistance. A client system might also be a couple in marital therapy that continues to practice abusive interactions between sessions, even though alternative interactions have been offered and practiced in therapy. Changing old and comfortable coping and communication patterns is threatening. The future is unknown to the client.

The therapist can provide significant emotional support to the client by recognizing ambivalence. Verbally acknowledging that change is hard, scary, and uncomfortable helps. Also, giving the resistance "back to the client" is an important method to diffuse rather than escalate resistance. Telling the client, "You're changing too much" or "You're proceeding too fast" or "There must be other, more important concerns that keep you from trying new things" or "Maybe the old way wasn't so bad after all" drops the pressure from the therapist and allows the client to reevaluate the desired area for growth.

THERAPIST'S RELUCTANCE TO INTERVENE

Many normal obstacles interfere with successful therapy, especially in the beginning. Central to removing these barriers is a willingness to learn from one's mistakes and be open to information. Supportive, safe, and "live data" supervision (using videotape or cotherapy) offers vital information in helping beginning therapists avoid problems and find a solid footing.

Sometimes trainees do not risk an intervention until everything is totally clear. Lack of experience and anxiety over dealing with presenting issues can result in gathering too much information or spending many sessions unfocused. Clients need to experience some progress early in the therapy—without this, they might not come back. One idea is to offer some therapeutic "gift" to the client early, even before the direction of therapy has been decided. These gifts include interventions such as normalizing, reframing, amplifying positive interactions in the family, or congratulating the family on their courage to seek help.

Also, after two to three sessions, the therapist may want to use the clinical reasoning process discussed in Chapter 5 to understand the presenting problems and to focus possible interventions. Once this is done, you just need to jump in and risk trying something.

THERAPIST–CLIENT AGENDA AND TIMING MISMATCH

Another key area of stuckness comes from a mismatch between the therapist's goals and the family's goals. Especially enthusiastic at the start of their work, family therapy practicum students often want to "change the world" and "fix" the family. The therapist–client mismatch becomes particularly clear when a therapist begins to direct the family toward something they don't want. For example, a 10-year-old child of a single mother is brought to therapy because of chronic lying at school and at home. The therapist focuses on the task of including the father, who has visited with the child only five times in her life, into solving the problem, and the mother doesn't return to therapy. When a therapist focuses more on a theoretical perspective or his or her own agenda rather than the working relationship with the client, a mismatch is more likely to occur.

Change can be achieved at several levels, referred to as first-order and second-order change. First-order change denotes behavioral change, that is, acting in new ways. Second-order change requires behavioral, cognitive, affective, and relational changes, that is, change within an entire system. It's important to determine what order of change the therapist and client system desire so that therapy is planned appropriately. Usually, struggles occur around the systemic differences of defining the "right kind of change." For example, a rigid, authoritarian parent may present his son for therapy because of problems with homework. After focusing on this presenting problem by bringing some flexibility into when and where the child does the homework, the parent terminates therapy. The therapist, however, wants to address the overall rigidity of the parental system during adolescence and wants to continue therapy to achieve more adaptability—for the entire family, and for the son's future growth. The parent requests first-order change, which is at odds with the therapist's desire to generate second-order change. The following case further illustrates the differences between these levels of change.

A 15-year-old girl is presented as the IP in her family. The current problem is her continuing to come home late in the evening, after her imposed curfew. The parents have attempted to change her behavior by first simply asking that she come home on time or call. The girl agreed, but continued to come home late. The parents then told her that if she was late one night, she would have to come home early the next night by the same amount of time. She agreed to try this but later said it was unfair, and that their curfew was too early to begin with.

In the therapy session, the parents were asked to talk about their concerns and feelings for their daughter. They also talked about their fears of her growing up and leaving them, and of their lack of contact with her friends. At one point the father said, "I just feel like I don't know who you are anymore." The girl disclosed some of her frustrations with her parents and some of the pressures she was under at school.

Although the problems were not immediately solved, the parents and their daughter were able to talk about their stresses and feelings about change in their relationship. They worked out a new approach to the problem of coming home late by discussing their individual perspectives on the problem and several possible solutions.

The parents' attempt to change the situation before coming to therapy was primarily to change the girl's behavior. First, they asked her to come home on time and then they tried to develop consequences for not coming in on time. These are examples of first-order change that is targeted at the behavioral level. In the therapy session, family members explored their relationships and feelings about each other. They also discussed concerns about the problem and about the changes they were facing. Ultimately, the changes that began to take place in the family's ability to communicate moved beyond behaviors. Changes slowly occurred on several levels, including the affective, relational, and behavioral domains, which will impact the entire family system. Thus, we have second-order change.

In addition to being clear about the level of change desired by client and therapist, timing of interventions must be considered. Family therapy highlights the need to be intentional about when certain tasks need to be done and who needs to be a part of the change. This concern is revisited throughout therapy. A remarried couple might need to solve differences and work on better communication skills before inviting an ex-wife to join in sessions concerning a college-age daughter. If the ex-wife was brought in before the remarried couple dealt with their own conflicts, a therapist might see resistance. The therapist must handle the important issues of matching agendas and timing to proceed effectively.

THERAPIST'S LACK OF THEORETICAL CLARITY

Another common therapist contribution to problems in the therapeutic process stems from a lack of clarity about one's theoretical perspective. Beginning therapists jump at the opportunity to translate what they've learned in class into a counseling session. After joining and assessment, the therapist might take a grab-bag approach to interventions. For example, John and Jean enter therapy after an argument in which they decide to call off their engagement. As high school sweethearts, they and their fairly enmeshed families have found increasing tension around wedding plans—styles and expectations differ. A therapist begins to work on the couple's communication and problem-solving skills during the first two working sessions, but then shifts to a structural perspective in order to more appropriately separate a mother–daughter alignment. In a subsequent session, we find the therapist encouraging the expression of grief. While none of these clinical interventions or understandings is incorrect, the therapist might begin to lose focus of the theoretical perspective, appropriate interventions for that theory, and therapeutic goals. When this happens, supervisors often hear practicum students say, "I'm lost."

Your theoretical orientation helps to define what domain of therapy is central to your work with a particular client. Affective, behavioral, cognitive, and/or relational domains may be affected. It's important for the therapist to keep in mind which of these domains therapy will affect. For example, in experiential therapies the domain of affect needs to be emphasized. Thus, a therapist might have difficulty debriefing a family sculpture that depicts a child's feeling "left out" when the family is one that doesn't readily allow for expression of sad feelings. Experiential therapy also requires family members to be in the therapy room in order for authentic and honest self-disclosure to be accomplished. It would be insufficient to address being "left out" if the child was not present. In contrast, from a strategic perspective where behavioral sequences are central, the parents of an oppositional adolescent son might resist "catching their child following the rules" when he does follow them. The son wouldn't necessarily need to be in the room in order to facilitate change in this family.

Therapists who are focused and intentional about what they offer to a family will help clients manage their resistance positively. Therapists who lose focus about therapeutic goals and domains of therapy (as addressed by their theoretical orientation) will frustrate both themselves and their clients. This process can be complicated when new therapists receive conflicting feedback from different supervisors, each with different therapeutic agendas. Just as different perspectives must be negotiated during therapy, so must the responsible therapist ascertain which supervision will be most beneficial for clinical work.

The most helpful way to stay on track in facilitating change is to set clear goals with the family during the first few sessions and then select theoretical perspectives that will best serve reaching those goals. A conscious blending of several theories is often appropriate; however, goals need to be prioritized—which are of first, second, or third importance? These issues should be handled by the therapist and family in the initial sessions at regular intervals. Without prioritizing the goals, session agendas are unclear for everyone.

SUPERVISION

Supervision can be one of the most important ways for you to get help on a case. Ideally, you will have access to a supervisor who has both strong clinical and supervisory skills. Individuals who are approved supervisors through the American Association for Marriage and Family Therapy (AAMFT) have received special instruction in supervision (including supervision of their supervision) and have a minimum of 2,000 hours of clinical experience.

Although the supervisor's qualifications are important, you must also be willing to do your part to make the supervision experience worthwhile. This requires that you be willing to share issues and cases that are a source of struggle for you. You need to be willing to seek live supervision or show videotapes of cases in which you feel stuck or frustrated. Therapists who only present cases in which they feel competent are missing an opportunity to grow and stretch themselves through supervision.

You must also be willing to give your supervisor feedback on what is needed from supervision. You might specify a particular issue you would like feedback on in a case, or you might indicate the need for more positive feedback if you are struggling with confidence issues. In some cases, you may need to tell your supervisor that the suggestions do not seem to fit the family, and explore with him or her why this is the case, which may lead to new, more helpful insights. Most supervisors will appreciate any feedback you can provide that gives a clearer sense of what is needed from supervision.

SELF-SUPERVISION QUESTIONS

In addition to getting supervision from a qualified supervisor, you should begin to develop your own self-supervision skills. In other words, you should develop self-reflective methods and questions that can be used in place of getting supervision from another individual. Watching videotapes of your own sessions is helpful in providing a more objective viewpoint on what happens in therapy. Often therapists who have watched their videotapes prior to receiving supervision will report gaining an important insight to their work.

You can also develop a list of self-supervision questions that are helpful when you get stuck in a case—a checklist of items that can frequently cause difficulties. A list of sample self-supervision questions are listed in Table 10.1. For example, a therapist who feels frustrated by the lack of movement in a case may discover upon going through the checklist of questions that he or she is working much harder than the clients. This in turn might lead the therapist to explore the clients' motivation for therapy or the possible negative consequences of change. Used in this manner, a checklist of questions can be an effective means of helping you trouble-shoot a case on your own.

PEER CONSULTATION

Consultation with other therapists can be important source of information. Consultation does not always need to be with more experienced therapists to be helpful. Other beginning therapists may be able to offer helpful insights simply because they provide a fresh or more objective perspective. Consulting with other therapists has the added benefit of providing a professional support system, which will help you avoid burnout. Similarly, professional groups and associations provide valuable networking opportunities, information, research, and support for therapists. Table 10.2 lists a number of organizations that provide links among professionals.

DOING A LITERATURE SEARCH

The marriage and family therapy literature is a rich source of information for dealing with difficult cases. Reading the literature is particularly helpful in cases where you have limited experience with a particular problem or population. For example, a therapist who has not worked with a couple experiencing infertility could read books or articles on the issues that infertile couples must face.

TABLE 10.1. Self-Supervision Questions

When feeling stuck or encountering client resistance, ask:

1. Am I, as the therapist, working harder than the clients?
2. What are negative consequences to change that my clients may be struggling with?
3. Does the problem serve some positive function or purpose?
4. Have I clearly assessed the client's goals, and does the client see me as working on those goals?
5. Have I sufficiently joined with the client?
6. Does the client see therapy or the therapist as credible?
7. Is my frustration a possible sign of my own personal issues interfering with the client's?
8. Are my reactions or responses isomorphic to the system?
9. Have I appropriately balanced the responsibility for change? (Or do I find myself siding with one person over the other?)
10. Have I identified two or three key therapeutic issues or themes, or am I trying to focus on too many things?

Each year new books are introduced that address both general clinical practice as well as specific problem areas or special populations. In addition, there are several professional journals devoted to marriage and family therapy. Table 10.3 provides a resource guide on comprehensive indexes and abstracts, as well as a list of relevant journals.

As the number of journals and books on family therapy steadily increases, the most effective strategy for tapping this rich resource is to do a literature search to investigate specific clinical problems and populations. Many comprehensive indexes or abstracts (e.g., *PsycLIT*) are on a computerized database, which makes doing a literature search easy and painless. By entering multiple keyword parameters, indexes such as *PsycLIT* can quickly be searched to provide a limited number of articles that would be of interest to the reader. For example, a therapist who is feeling stuck in treating an adolescent with depression could search the literature using keywords such as "depression" and "adolescents."

DEALING WITH CANCELLATIONS AND "NO SHOWS"

A 19-year-old client who has been coming to therapy for depression missed an appointment because he had a job interview; he forgot to call the therapist and cancel the appointment. A younger adolescent client failed to make her morning appointment because she overslept, and she blamed her

TABLE 10.2. Professional Organizations

American Association for Marriage and Family Therapy
1100 17th Street NW
Washington, DC 20036

National Council on Family Relations
1219 University Avenue SE
Minneapolis, MN 55414

American Psychological Association
(Division 43, Family Psychology Section)
750 First Street NE
Washington, DC 20002–4242

Association for Advancement of Behavior Therapy
15 West 36th Street
New York, NY 10018

Society for Psychotherapy Research
21 Bloomingdale Road
White Plains, NY 10605

American Family Therapy Association
2020 Pennsylvania Avenue NW, Suite 273
Washington, DC 20006

International Association for Marriage and
Family Counselors
American Counseling Association
5999 Stevenson Avenue
Alexandria, VA 22304–3300

Society for Research in Child Development
University of Chicago
5720 Woodlawn Avenue
Chicago, IL 60637

Society of Teachers of Family Medicine
8880 Ward Parkway
P.O. Box 8729
Kansas City, MO 64114

mother for not waking her up. A family being treated for anxiety in two children begins canceling and rescheduling appointments until 4 weeks have gone by without a session.

Cancellations and missed appointments offer important information to the therapist and must be acknowledged and evaluated. Since systemic thinking assumes a relational nature to therapeutic work, cancellations and missed appointments need to be interpreted relationally. Therapists need to respond to both, usually by telephone, to determine the meaning

TABLE 10.3. Resource Guide: Indexes and Abstracts; Professional Journals

Indexes and abstracts

Family studies

Child Development Abstracts and Bibliography
Chicago: University of Chicago Press, for the Society for Research in Child Development. Contains abstracts from professional periodicals and reviews books related to the growth and development of children. Issued three times a year. Includes author and subject indexes.

Family Studies Database
Baltimore, MD: National Information Services. Indexes over 800 journals on a quarterly basis.

Sage Family Studies Abstracts
Thousand Oaks, CA: Sage. Indexes journals, books, pamphlets, government publications, significant speeches, legislative research studies, and other "fugitive material." Includes author and subject indexes. Issued quarterly.

Social sciences

Sociological Abstracts
San Diego, CA: Sociological Abstracts. Issued bimonthly with cumulative annual indexes. Abstracts the world's serial literature in sociology and related disciplines. Includes subject, author, and source indexes. Also contains a supplement, *International Review of Publications in Sociology.*

Social Sciences Citation Index
Philadelphia: Institute for Scientific Information. A citation index covering several thousand journals. Is a multidisciplinary index to the worldwide literature of the social sciences. Each multivolume edition contains sciences. Each edition contains four separate but interrelated parts: citation index, permuterm subject index, corporate index, and source index.

Psychological Abstracts
Washington, DC: American Psychological Association. Consists of nonevaluative summaries of the world's journal and book literature in psychology and related disciplines. Includes subject and author indexes.

Journals in Psychology
Washington, DC: American Psychological Association. Index of journals of the psychological sciences. Indexed both by subject matter and journal.

Women's studies

Studies on Women Abstracts
Abingdon, Oxfordshire, UK: Carfax. International abstracting of journals and books in the main areas of women's studies. Includes author and subject indexes.

Women Studies Abstracts
New Brunswick, NJ: Transaction. Subject index to articles on women studies. Issued quarterly with annual author and subject indexes appearing in the fourth issue.

(cont.)

TABLE 10.3. (cont.)

Professional journals

Family psychotherapy periodicals

American Journal of Orthopsychiatry
Australian and New Zealand Journal of Family Therapy
California Therapist
Contemporary Family Therapy
Dulwich Centre Newsletter
Family Process
Family Therapy
Family Therapy Networker
Journal of Couples Therapy
Journal of Divorce and Remarriage
Journal of Family Psychology
Journal of Family Psychotherapy
Journal of Family Therapy
Journal of Feminist Family Therapy
Journal of Marital and Family Therapy
Journal of Systemic Therapies

Family periodicals

Family Relations
Families in Society
Journal of Comparative Family Studies
Journal of Family History
Journal of Family Issues
Journal of Marriage and the Family
Marriage and Family Review

Psychotherapy periodicals

Clinical Psychology Review
Journal of Sex and Marital Therapy
Psychotherapy

Psychology periodicals

Advances in Behaviour Research and Therapy
Advances in Descriptive Psychology
American Journal of Psychology
American Psychologist
Annual Review of Psychology
APA Monitor
Behavioral and Brain Sciences
Behavioral Science
British Journal of Psychology
Clinical Psychologist
Contemporary Psychology
Human Behavior
Humanitas

(cont.)

TABLE 10.3. (cont.)

Journal of Abnormal and Social Psychology
Journal of Applied Psychology
Journal of Consulting and Clinical Psychology
Journal of Experimental Psychology
Journal of Health and Social Behavior
Journal of Personality
Journal of Psychology and Theology
Journal of Sex Research
Journal of the Experimental Analysis of Behavior
Law and Psychology Review
Mind
New Directions in Psychology
Psychological Bulletin
Psychological Review
Psychology

Family medicine periodicals

American Family Physician
Family and Community Health
Family Practice Research Journal
Journal of Family Practice

---

of the "no show" or cancellation. Sometimes the meaning is quite concrete and practical: It's simply a missed appointment—"I had a flat tire and couldn't get it fixed in time for our appointment." It's useful to review one's policy on cancellations and missed appointments at this time and to clarify any misunderstandings. Most agencies and practices have a 24-hour cancellation policy in which clients are billed for the appointment unless they cancel at least 24 hours before the appointment. This policy may be waived for emergencies; however, "emergency" must be defined.

"No shows" or cancellations can indicate a reevaluation of the therapeutic process itself. Evaluating goals needs to be done throughout the therapeutic process, preferably with the clients' involvement. But when clients have difficulty with this, they might communicate their discomfort by canceling or missing appointments. For example, a couple comes to therapy to decrease the number of fights they have. This goal is partially addressed by encouraging solid communication skills such as "I" messages and active listening. After a bit of relief, the couple starts canceling or consistently rescheduling their appointments. The therapist requests a reevaluation session to discuss if therapy has satisfied the couple's goals and could be terminated, if appointments might be set at more infrequent intervals, or if other goals need to be addressed. It's important to set a collaborative tone to the re-evaluation process since client and therapist goals might not match.

Cancellations and "no shows" might also indicate that parts of the client system are questioning the therapeutic process. For example, as a depressed adolescent begins to speak more assertively about his needs, perhaps even yell sometimes, the rest of the family might wonder if therapy is doing any good, since this "isn't the behavior we wanted." Cancellations and missed appointments can simply indicate the system's ambivalence about change.

"No shows" and cancellations might also be a result of a disruption in the therapeutic alliance. This is particularly true for clients with certain family of origin issues, such as abandonment, or with Axis II DSM-IV diagnoses, such as borderline or avoidant personality disorders. Some clients might be extremely sensitive to a therapist's taking sides during a family session, experiencing the therapist's validation of another family member as invalidating them. Clients express this indirectly by not showing for an appointment or by "forgetting." Again, depending on the therapist's theoretical orientation, this aspect of the client's reaction will be explored in more or less depth. All therapists need to determine, on an ongoing basis, the solidity of the therapeutic alliance in order to proceed successfully in therapy.

Cancellations and missed appointments also result from "constraints" to change presented by many clients, especially those who are socially and economically disadvantaged. Such actions might simply have to do with choices between paying for therapy and paying for groceries or rent. Also, lack of access to transportation can constrain one's ability to attend therapy. It's important to be sensitive to these realistic constraints and to negotiate ways of increasing resources to keep therapy accessible. There's nothing magic about scheduling therapy once a week. This format stems from early analytic patterns of scheduling three to five sessions each week. Systemic interventions can be creatively managed, as highlighted by some of the Italian family therapists (the Milan group) who might do several hours of intensive family work and then not see the family for several months.

The key is that the therapist participates actively in understanding the meaning of the "no show" or cancellation and manages this meaning therapeutically.

DIFFICULTY GETTING OTHER FAMILY MEMBERS TO THERAPY

The family members who do not make it into treatment may be absent for several different reasons. The first area to investigate is communication between family members. Were they asked to be a part of therapy? How was this discussed? Sometimes therapy can be viewed as another issue to fight about, and it becomes the problem rather than a vehicle for solving problems. Each family member makes a choice in coming or not coming to therapy, exercising some power in the family's decision-making process. If a family member is involved in a power struggle, it may be helpful for the therapist to intervene as a mediator to invite the member to come to the session. Offering to make telephone contact with a reluctant client can help to serve as a bridge to therapy.

Family members may not come in because they don't think that they have a problem. It's not unusual for one member of a couple to want to go to therapy while the other is reluctant or ambivalent. The reluctant partner often feels that he or she does not really have a problem, so "why should I go?" It can be useful for the therapist to indicate to this partner that he or she has a valuable perspective and pertinent information to offer, regardless of who appears to have the problem. Further, the therapist might point out to the reluctant client that he or she is in the best position to relay his or her own story. Absence might cause his or her voice may go unheard or his or her position to be misrepresented.

Some family members may be reluctant to attend sessions due to their discomfort with others in the family. In some situations it may be useful to first work with subsystems and join effectively with them before bringing in all of the family members at once. In some families, being together and having direct communication is a rarity and may need to be "worked up to" on a gradual basis over several sessions.

Reluctant clients may be skeptical of the value of therapy or they may have had a previous negative experience in therapy. Their previous experiences and views about therapy should be explored and understood. It can be helpful to suggest that the client only commit initially to one visit. This session should provide an opportunity for the person to be heard as well as a chance to hear what other family members have to say. The focus of this session will likely be on providing a safe place for communication and not on making changes.

HANDLING SECRETS

Some therapists prefer the "clarity" of individual therapy, which simplifies the clinical contract. However, systemically oriented therapists understand that involving more than one person is a powerful resource in the change process. With this power comes the issue of confidentiality and the potential problem of secrecy. Most important for the systemically oriented therapist to understand and avoid is the easy trap of collusion, or re-creating the same relational dynamics that brought the clients into therapy in the first place.

The following example illustrates how collusion can develop. An anxious client calls you to make an appointment for therapy in order to talk about her husband. You schedule the appointment with her alone and listen to her story, which includes news that she's been having an affair with a family friend for the past 5 months. She thinks her lover is going to end the relationship and she's very uncertain as to what to do next. "Part of me wants to make my marriage work, of course, but my husband can't know about the affair, so I want you to promise not to tell him when I bring him in for some marital counseling." If the therapist quickly reassures the client that information is confidential and then begins therapy without addressing the impact of the secret, collusion has occurred. More importantly, the therapist has given over an important domain of powerful information to the client, without coparticipating in defining how the secret might affect clinical work. Like resistance, collusion will occur. The therapist, however, must determine and actively participate in the control of pertinent information. Without this, the therapist is working with one arm tied behind his or her back.

Some therapists manage this dilemma by not allowing any confidential information to be disclosed—all sessions are with all family members and any phone contact will be disclosed in the next therapy session. Some therapists respect the confidential nature of information and determine that sometimes they will hold the confidence providing it doesn't interfere with therapeutic work. Some family therapy theories would say that secrets are mostly powerful in a negative way. Bowenian theory might see secrets as helping to create pathology in a subsequent generation; therefore, disclosing any secret would be therapeutic. Other theories, such as emotionally focused therapy, might be less interested in how truth was managed in the past and wholly interested in the honest sharing of emotional and behavioral information within the therapy session.

Again, one's clarity of theoretical focus as well as what is needed to maintain the therapeutic alliance must be evaluated in order to manage family secrets constructively.

HOW AGENCIES CONTRIBUTE TO BEING STUCK

Although family therapy has gained visibility and respect over the past several decades, it's a relatively new kid on the block within the mental health world. Agencies and institutions have developed to serve the needs of individuals, but they need to adapt to accommodate the different epistemology of systems thinking. For example, does the agency allow a therapist to keep a "family file" or does each family member need to be assessed individually—that is, given a diagnosis or mental status exam? Does the agency have senior supervisors familiar with the theory and practice of family therapy? Practically, do the rooms of the agency provide enough space or evening and weekend office hours to serve the needs of the family? Without considering these concerns, an agency's organization might interfere with effective treatment of the whole family.

Beginning family therapists need to be aware of the agency's level of commitment to systems-oriented therapy before beginning their work. In this way, expectations and change can be facilitated positively. As in doing good therapy, know who is supportive of family therapy, explore their position within the agency as a whole, and enter the system respectful of its power base. When significant change is needed, be willing to serve as a helpful partner in that change, perhaps by offering to review and edit intake forms. Offer your own perspective about the cases you observe or nondefensively ask for feedback regarding alternative theoretical positions, after explaining how you're dealing with a case. Find family therapy supports outside the agency if you're working as a Lone Ranger (even he had Tonto).

Interestingly, the most resistant cases appear when all systems involved—client, therapist, and agency—get stuck together. This is called isomorphism, a reference to the creation of similar relational structures across several systems. Client therapist and supervisory systems exist from the beginning of therapy. Since systems tend to re-create themselves at several levels, and beginning therapists are accountable across several systems, at times problems at one system level can be observed at another level. For example, a wife presented the problem of feeling powerless to change her husband; the therapist tried several interventions to help her respond differently to her husband, but she continued to do things in the same style; the supervisor directed the therapist to utilize another modality of therapy with this woman, but the therapist wanted to stay with the current agenda for a few more sessions. What we see at these three system levels is isomorphism, or similar interactional styles developing across systems. Isomorphism sometimes can be positive, but it also can signal areas of stuckness in the therapeutic relationship. Consider the case of Carl, a family therapist, and his client Bob. Carl has some difficulties in his work setting, which in turn have a direct effect on Bob's process of recovery.

Bob, a 32-year-old Caucasian male, reluctantly admits himself to an inpatient substance abuse program. His wife has been threatening to divorce him, and his employer indicates that Bob's work performance has suffered due to his alcohol-related absences. Bob feels that he drinks recreationally and can handle his problems. He does agree that he shouldn't drink so much during the week and thinks he can control it. He has even "quit completely several times, for 2 or 3 months." He thinks his wife should be more understanding of the stress that he's under because of his work and concentrate on her own problems. His fear of losing his job and his wife motivate him enough to enter a treatment program. His presentation is sarcastic, and he's resentful that he has to be there. He says that he'll stay for awhile because he promised his wife. When asked about his goals he says, "I'm still trying to figure out why I'm here and who is in charge."

Bob's therapist is Carl, a 40-year-old Caucasian marriage and family therapist and a recovering alcoholic who has been working in the substance abuse field for the past 7 years. He has been sober for 12 years. Carl is a very committed professional who believes in combining the 12-step program with psychotherapy in order to help clients achieve sobriety. He works long hours and gets a great deal of satisfaction from his job. He feels that he has a realistic picture of what can be accomplished in treatment given "the time limits and nature of the disease of alcoholism."

Carl has worked with many clients like Bob who present an initial high degree of resistance to treatment and "denial as to the extent of their problem." Carl expects that Bob's hostility will begin to dissipate once he gets involved in some group meetings and begins to accept his problems.

In their first meeting, some of Bob's anger is directed at Carl. Bob insists that Carl can't really understand him and that he is only interested in keeping him in the hospital so that he can keep his job. Carl's response is to maintain his distance from Bob's anger and ask Bob further questions about his feelings about being in treatment. This helps to stop the attacks, but Bob continues to be fairly hostile throughout the session. In their second session Bob talks about his initial group meeting. He begins with sarcastic comments about some of the members and talks about why he doesn't think he belongs there. Further questions by the therapist help to identify some of Bob's feelings of identification with two of the group members who feel ambivalent about the treatment process. Carl's questions throughout the remainder of the session help Bob to disclose some of his fears about treatment. Carl leaves the second session feeling as though he has begun to develop a therapeutic alliance with Bob and the treatment process has begun.

Bob's treatment progresses well during his first week in treatment. He has quickly begun to like and respect Carl and is making good use of the treatment process. Carl also feels good about Bob's progress and begins to cautiously self-disclose about his own battle with alcohol. Carl sees some of himself in Bob, so he finds it a bit easier to talk with him than with most of the patients.

Toward the end of the Bob's first week in treatment Carl begins to have some difficulties with his supervisor and some of the facility's policies. There has been a growing amount of required paperwork. The hospital has become more restrictive about overtime and has developed policies to discourage it. Carl's supervisor feels that his work with the patients is good but that his documentation is not up to par and he must improve in this area. Carl feels that his supervisor is more concerned about protecting his job than providing quality care, and he the supervisor have a heated argument over this issue.

In his next meeting with Bob, Carl is still upset about his meeting with his supervisor. Although he knows better, he begins to talk about some of his frustrations with the hospital and his job. This becomes the discussion of most of the session. Bob is very interested in Carl's difficulties with his job and asks lots of questions. Toward the end of the session he indicates that he has had some of the same kind of problems with his boss.

At his next group meeting, Bob announces that he's going to leave the treatment program. He says he has learned that the program "doesn't have its priorities straight" and he doesn't "belong there."

The key for a beginning therapist, or any therapist, is to recognize when an isomorphic process is occurring. Unchecked, isomorphisms can be detrimental to therapy. With recognition comes the ability to be a more effective agent of change for the client.

COUNTERTRANSFERENCE: HOW THERAPIST'S ISSUES INTERFERE

Sharon was a 25-year-old intern who had been working comfortably with latency- and teenage youngsters at a family service agency. One afternoon, Sharon met with the mother of a 7-year-old female client. The woman was very critical of the child and had unrealistic expectations of her daughter. Sharon thought the mother was expecting the girl to be "perfect," and she felt protective of the child. She identified with the little girl and noticed that the mother's criticism and demands reminded her of her relationship with her mother. Recognizing this connection, Sharon was able to disengage from a power struggle with the mother and maintain her composure through the rest of the session. Later, she sought supervision and was able to get help in separating her reactions to the client's mother from those toward her own mother.

These processes, which regularly come into play in therapy, stem from what analytically oriented therapists term "transference" and "countertransference." Often ignored or relabeled in family therapy texts, they relate to a phenomenon that is often discussed in supervision. Family therapy, in its attempt to establish its own specialization separate from psychoanalytic roots, tends to be more technique-focused and less concerned about the therapeutic relationship. More recent writings in family therapy, such as narrative therapy, have asked important questions concerning the interpersonal context of therapy. Certainly, it is in the interpersonal arena that self and family are shaped.

In very simple terms, "transference" denotes the interpersonal material brought into the therapeutic relationship by the client, and "countertransference" denotes the interpersonal material brought into the therapeutic relationship by the therapist. Object relations theories understand these components as the essential working domain for therapy, since in transference the client offers a re-creation of the affective, behavioral, and cognitive issues that need to be reworked for positive growth to take place. Countertransference, too, must be internally monitored and interpersonally utilized for therapeutic progress to occur.

Whatever terms are used, part of the process of therapy (especially when it lasts for some time) involves the way feelings, behaviors, and cognitions from the past are played out in the current therapeutic setting. For example, a single mother comes into therapy for treatment of her depression. After several weeks of work in which the therapist empathizes with her situation and encourages access to underutilized resources in her life, she becomes more quiet and occasionally says, "I know you're going to get mad at me, but. . . ." The client expects the therapist will react to her just as her own mother had—with criticism and disappointment at her lack of progress.

Feelings, thoughts, and behaviors also emerge from the therapist's past. Almost weekly, in supervising practicum students, we hear the words, "I thought I had my father (or mother, or boyfriend, or "ex") in the room with me during part of the session."

In managing transference and countertransference, it is important first to normalize personal reactions during therapy. Note that these phenomena will probably occur more often when doing individual therapy than when doing couple or family work, because in the latter, several persons can serve the purpose of projective identification, that is, expecting someone other than the therapist to act as someone significant from one's own background.

Second, several common, though varied, themes can be understood in this process, including helplessness, control, and sexuality. Most often these themes develop when there's some form of anxiety in the system—a normal reaction to any change process. Some clients present with a "help me" cry that seems stronger than "I need help"; these clients readily stay in a victim stance even when they're no longer being victimized. A common therapist reaction is to feel overwhelmed by the client. For example, one intern remarked, "I found myself making phone calls to this family and worrying about them before I went to sleep at night. They were all-consuming."

We do have many clients in this work who are in great pain and need, and compassionate reactions must be a part of what we do. However, good therapy requires that a working relationship be established in which each member of the system shares in therapy's progress. Without this working alliance, a client might remain stuck as a victim and the therapist will be "burnt out" by the client system. Clarifying each client's responsibility for the therapy will need to be reviewed if the helplessness theme continues.

A control issue is present when one member of the system demands or dictates to everyone where the therapy should or should not go. If the client initiates control, then commonly the therapist feels criticized or incompetent. Young therapists, in particular, often look for approval from their clients as a way to feel adequate. Working with a demanding and critical client can distract the therapist from the job of facilitating change within the entire system. Further, the therapist might be pulled to react as other family members have acted, perhaps passively. It's important for the therapist to know his or her limits and actively acknowledge them. Beginning therapists need to feel comfortable about stating they are just that—beginning. As long as the therapist is backed up by solid, supportive supervision, this is fairly easy to do.

Therapists can inadvertently contribute to this controlling theme. Feeling internal pressure to be "in charge" may undermine a therapist's ability to share with clients the responsibility for doing the work necessary for change. Also, paradoxically, controlling persons need to be "reframed" as the most vulnerable or out of control. Controlling persons often are highly needy individuals and must be treated with care. If a therapist discovers that this is his or her style it would be critical to examine the roots of this attitude in order to facilitate a more therapeutic alignment with the family.

The third theme is sexuality. Particularly in opposite-gender therapeutic relationships, romantic or erotic messages may be verbally or nonverbally introduced into the session. Therapists might be attracted or scared by this. Many interns have disclosed that they have sexual dreams about their clients. Several important aspects of the sexuality theme can be noted. First, gender issues are a part of all human relationships; this can't be avoided. Further, some people sexualize these gender factors, especially when they have been abused or are needy in this area. Finally, the emotional legacy from one's family of origin influences how comfortably or uncomfortably this domain will be addressed within the therapeutic relationship.

As a general rule, seeking therapy or peer consultation must be a part of professional development no matter how much experience one has. Therapy will be "loaded" if one's family of origin issues touch the clients with whom one works. All therapists have an "Achilles' heel" in their work, but utilizing vulnerable parts of ourselves in our work can enhance and enrich the therapy greatly.

Finally, recognizing what type of work one does well, given certain family of origin experiences, provides a solid focus for one's energies. Learning about oneself is a lifelong journey, and this profession provides a wonderful context for continuing down this path.

OTHER PERSONAL INFLUENCES

Feeling Burned Out

At first glance, one would not anticipate that someone who is just beginning a career as a family therapist would experience feelings of burnout. Yet the fact is that many beginning therapists experience some degree of burnout because of several factors.

First, learning to do therapy can be demanding. Worrying about one's competence as a beginning therapist can take its toll over time, perhaps diminishing some of the enjoyment of doing therapy. Beginning therapists may also overextend themselves or worry excessively about their clients until they learn to better manage their emotional boundaries.

Second, therapists have other stressors outside of their clinical work. For example, you may have other classes, comprehensive exams, or a master's or doctoral thesis to complete as part of your training program. You may need to work to pay for school or living expenses, or may have a family or partner who needs your time and energy. You may experience considerable stress from trying to successfully meet all these commitments.

Third, the courses or clinical work may raise personal issues for you as you learn to do therapy. Insights gained from clinical training inevitably lead student therapists to reexamine their own lives and families. Although this process can become the catalyst for significant personal growth, it can also place one more additional demand on the beginning therapist.

In order to avoid burnout, you need to build in time for "charging your batteries." Individuals who are faced with extreme time demands often put off taking personal time to do this. Taking time for yourself seems counterintuitive when faced with an overwhelming number of tasks to accomplish, but the time lost is often made up by being able to work with renewed energy and efficiency. Ironically, many therapists are willing to give this advice to their clients but have difficulty following it themselves.

Being willing to set limits is another important tool to avoid burnout. Beginning therapists often report setting their client schedule based largely on the convenience of their clients. In some cases, beginning therapists come in 5 days a week even though their case load only requires 3 or

4 days. As therapists gain experience, they often will become more willing to set some limits on their availability, giving them some protected time for themselves.

You also need a strong social support network. Many of us owe our families a great deal of credit for the emotional and/or financial support they provided during our training. However, you also need support and understanding that others who are not therapists cannot always provide. Both experienced and inexperienced therapists need colleagues with whom they can share clinical experiences to avoid burnout.

A Final Reminder

Finding oneself stuck, for whatever reason, in the midst of the therapeutic process is ubiquitous in the early stages of one's work. This chapter has identified some of the most common places therapists encounter challenges, and we've talked about ways to become "unstuck." Heightening awareness and developing specific skills and steps to take when we meet obstacles is an essential part of our work.

While dealing with particular challenges, it's important to keep the "big picture" in mind and recall that every point of stuckness provides a chance to increase competence and confidence. For example, learning to do therapy can be a strong catalyst for personal growth. What one learns about helping other families can be applied to one's own life and family, making it more enriching. Often the clients whom we struggle the most to help are the ones who give us the greatest sense of fulfillment when they actually do succeed in changing. As a therapist, you will be privileged to witness deeply moving moments of courage and compassion on the part of your clients, but as you move through the rough spots, it can be helpful to keep the following "reminders" at hand:

1. *Becoming a therapist takes time.* This is an opportunity for you to be a learner; you are not expected to be an expert. Becoming an effective therapist takes several years of training.
2. *Make sure you take care of yourself.* Utilize constructive means for stress reduction. Develop resources for support from other students, peers, and colleagues.
3. *Self-doubts are normal.* Be patient with yourself, focus on the positive, and pay attention to the developmental tasks of becoming a therapist.
4. *Use the skills that brought you to the field.* While you are learning lots of new theory and material, continue to pay attention to your intuition, your desire to work with others, and your natural abilities.

11

Termination

An important part of therapy is termination, even though it does not receive much attention in the literature; this is comparable to learning how to drive but never learning how to properly park the car and turn off the engine. A successful termination to therapy can be important for several reasons.

Terminations can be an effective way of empowering both the clients and the therapist. A successful termination should consolidate or reinforce the therapeutic gains of the client. For those who need to be referred or transferred, a successful termination can increase the likelihood that they will have a productive experience with a new therapist. For you as the therapist, a successful termination can help you understand how you were most helpful to the client, thereby building your confidence.

Terminations can also be important because they bring closure to the therapist–client relationship, an especially vital consideration in cases where the client and therapist have developed a strong connection over time. If properly handled, terminations can help clients and therapists deal with losses associated with ending the therapeutic relationship.

This chapter will discuss three types of terminations: client terminations, therapist terminations, and mutual terminations. Client terminations occur when the client unilaterally decides that therapy is over, whereas therapist terminations happen when the therapist unilaterally decides therapy should be discontinued. Mutual terminations occur when both the client and therapist agree on the termination, which typically occurs when both feel that client goals have been achieved.

Although these terminations will be discussed as three distinct phenomena, it is perhaps more accurate to view them on a continuum. Client and therapist terminations could be considered the two ends of the continuum, with mutual terminations representing the midpoint. Therefore, the therapeutic considerations outlined under each type may also partially apply to others, depending upon the situation.

MUTUAL TERMINATIONS

Most therapists strive for mutual terminations, which both you and your client are in agreement that the issues have been properly resolved and that continuing therapy is no longer necessary. In rare cases, both you and your client may agree that therapy should no longer be continued, but not necessarily because the issues are resolved. In one such example, both the therapist and client agreed that the client should discontinue therapy until she had finished a particularly difficult semester since most of her energy was devoted to finishing her studies. The client resumed therapy after completing her semester and had more energy to devote to her personal growth at that time.

When to Terminate

Although clients will sometimes bring up the topic of termination, it is often the therapist who must initiate a discussion about ending therapy (Fisch et al., 1985). Therefore, it is important that you recognize when it is time to begin termination.

Mutual terminations generally result from having successfully achieved the therapy goals. If these have been clearly identified and operationalized, then it will be easier you to recognize when to terminate (Fisch et al., 1985). In cases where goals are difficult to operationalize and define, you may need to rely on other indicators. If your clients have difficulty finding issues to discuss in therapy, this is often a sign that therapy is close to ending. Likewise, if you and your clients spend a lot of time in session in nontherapeutic talk or social chatter, termination should be considered.

One of the difficulties that can arise when considering termination with couples or families is that not all family members may feel equally ready for terminating therapy. Sometimes this is simply due to family members having different levels of confidence in their ability to handle problems as they arise without the therapist's guidance. Usually the most effective approach is to space out the sessions until all family members have developed the confidence to end therapy.

In other cases, family members may not be in agreement about terminating therapy because they have different expectations about what they want to achieve through therapy. In these cases, you are faced with the same dilemma as when clients enter therapy with different expectations. It is often possible for you to help the couple or family achieve some compromise. In one case, a couple had made significant changes in eliminating their high level of conflict. The husband reported being satisfied with the changes that had been made, and expressed interest in discontinuing therapy. While the wife agreed that the relationship was much improved, particularly in terms of the original goal of reducing conflict, she also expressed a desire to continue in therapy to improve the couple's sexual intimacy. A compromise was reached wherein the couple contracted to work on improving their sexual intimacy, but agreed to come to therapy every other week rather than weekly, as they had previously done.

Termination Goals

In terminating therapy, it's helpful to keep three goals in mind. The first is to help clients consolidate the gains they have made through therapy. Termination should reinforce the new skills, behaviors, or ways of thinking that the clients have learned.

The second goal of termination is to empower clients, giving them greater confidence in their ability to manage their issues on their own in the future. Another result of empowerment is that there will be a leveling of power between the therapist and the clients, reducing the clients' dependence on you and increasing self-reliance.

The third goal is to be sensitive to loss issues associated with terminations. Many clients develop a close relationship with their therapist and feel a sense of loss about ending the relationship. This is most likely to occur when you have worked with an individual, although at times couples or even families may have this experience. The sense of loss may be particularly keen for an individual who has a limited social support network to compensate for the loss of the therapeutic relationship.

Like clients, you may also experience a sense of loss when terminating therapy with certain clients. Therapists sometimes develop a very strong connection with certain clients, triggering feelings of sadness that the relationship is ending. These feelings can be compounded by other losses you may be experiencing. For example, when they leave their training program, many beginning therapists report sadness about ending relationships not only with clients that they care about, but also with colleagues and friends, by virtue of graduation. You need to be prepared to acknowledge and deal with these feelings as they arise.

Termination as Process

Terminations are more successful if they are conceptualized as a process rather than an event. When viewed from this perspective, termination is not confined to the final session but is a process that ideally begins earlier. In fact, one could argue that the goals for termination should be in the therapist's mind from the initial session. A therapist who is aware that a client has a very limited support network could anticipate that the client is likely to develop a strong dependence on him or her. This in turn will make termination a more acute loss for the client. In fact, clients who are overly dependent upon their therapist may manufacture problems to prolong the therapeutic relationship. Therefore, a therapist in this case would be wise to help the client develop a stronger support network during therapy. This will not only empower the client by giving him or her more resources, but will reduce the feelings of loss since the client will have others to turn to for emotional support.

Therapeutic Interventions in Termination

You can use several interventions to help achieve the goals for termination. One common intervention is to begin spacing out sessions. This strategy can give your clients time to consolidate the gains they have made, and also begins to build clients' confidence that they are managing problems on their own, since they have less contact with you.

In helping clients consolidate what they have gained from therapy, a number of questions can be asked. You can request that clients articulate what has changed for them and what they believe accounts for the change, or you can put them in the expert role by highlighting how successful they have been in addressing the problem and asking them for advice on how to work with other clients who have a similar difficulty. This approach has the advantage of empowering your clients in addition to helping them consolidate therapeutic gains. When asking clients to indicate what has brought about the changes, it's important that you give them permission to acknowledge things that may have happened outside of therapy. Some clients have difficulty answering the question of what they are doing differently. One possible approach to this problem is to ask them what they could do to make things worse, which often gives them insights into what positive changes have occurred (Hoffman, 1981). In other cases, you may need to help punctuate for your clients the changes they have made.

It's often helpful to clients to predict temporary relapses. Clients can be told that change is a matter of "two steps forward and one step back." This helps them be less threatened by temporary setbacks, which in turn provides greater confidence in managing problems on their own.

Clients respond very positively when you can share something special that they have taught you. This is an effective way to empower your clients, making them feel the relationship has been reciprocal. For example, one therapist told a couple how a particular metaphor that had emerged out of their work together had been helpful in his work with other clients. Like any intervention in therapy, the therapist must be sincere and not simply manufacture something.

Some therapists also like to give small gifts to clients to mark termination. The gifts should be of little monetary value so clients do not feel obligated to give a gift in return; rather, the gift should be rich in symbolic meaning. One therapist gave a couple an onion to symbolize the different layers they had explored and the emotions that therapy elicited. The onion provided a focal point for the therapist and couple to process the end of an important relationship. The gift could also be a reminder of an important therapeutic theme.

Special Issues in Termination

One special issue that can arise at termination is whether or not to accept gifts from clients. Some therapists believe they should not accept any gifts from clients under any circumstances. Others believe that it's permissible to accept gifts from clients provided they aren't expensive. The advantage of not accepting any gifts is that you are never placed in the position of having to decide if a gift is too expensive to accept. The disadvantage of refusing to accept a gift is that it may hurt the client's feelings, particularly if the gift was meant to be a symbolic gesture. Therapists who are willing to accept gifts must weigh the monetary and symbolic meaning of the gift. This makes the judgment more difficult, but gives you more options in how to respond. Each therapist must make a personal choice on which philosophy they will adopt regarding gifts from clients.

Another issue that can arise at termination are clients who would like to continue to have a relationship with you outside of therapy. We recommended that you avoid this situation. It is not uncommon for clients to return to therapy because of new problems that arise. If you begin a relationship with your clients after termination and they need to resume therapy, it puts you in the uncomfortable position of having a dual relationship with them. Therefore, a major reason to avoid a relationship after termination is to preserve your clients' right to return to therapy if needed.

Avoiding relationships outside of therapy not only protects the clients, but it can also protect you. If problems arise in the relationship outside of therapy for any reason, you are vulnerable to having your professional behavior questioned. A therapist who gets romantically involved with a client after terminating therapy could be accused of taking advantage of the client if the relationship sours.

Finally, another issue that therapists sometimes face are clients who do not wish to terminate, but who would like to continue therapy on a less frequent basis. Some therapists see this request as a sign that the client is too dependent upon the therapist. Other therapists believe that this arrangement is completely appropriate and desirable for some clients. Some therapists advocate booster sessions to help maintain treatment gains.

When clients request to continue therapy, you should carefully evaluate the motivation behind the request. The request may indeed signal excessive dependence upon you, particularly if your clients request seeing you on a frequent basis (more than once or twice a month). These clients typically have few people other than their therapist with whom they feel closely connected. You may then want to help your clients develop their support network to reduce their dependence on you.

However, the request to continue therapy doesn't always signal dependency issues. Some clients want to see their therapist periodically to help keep their family relationships healthy. For these clients, therapy is like going to the dentist for a 6-month preventative checkup. Other clients genuinely want to continue to grow, and they see therapy as a way to facilitate that growth. Therapy assumes more of a coaching or mentoring role, rather than a crisis or problem-solving role. Therefore, a therapist could feel comfortable seeing these clients periodically as a preventative measure or to facilitate the clients' desires for continued growth. For example, one of the authors (L. W.) continued to see a couple once every 3 months to facilitate the couple's continued growth and enrichment of their relationship.

THERAPIST TERMINATIONS

There will be times when a therapist may unilaterally decide therapy should be discontinued. Like client terminations, there can be a variety of reasons leading to a therapist termination. A common reason is that you are moving or terminating employment with an agency. In some instances, a therapist may wish to end therapy with particular clients due to specific issues in the case. The therapist may feel unqualified to deal with the issues, or feel that personal issues interfere with the case.

You might also suggest terminating therapy if agreement cannot be reached on the therapeutic contract or you strongly suspect the clients are not ready for change. However, you should work closely with these clients to make termination of therapy as much of a mutual decision as possible. In one case, for example, a therapist felt it was necessary to address the husband's severe mistrust of his wife as part of the couple's dynamics. However, the husband never agreed with the therapist's assessment that this was an important issue to address, creating an impasse in therapy. The therapist discussed with the couple how the lack of agreement on this key issue probably precluded a successful outcome to therapy. The couple agreed, resulting in a mutual decision to terminate therapy and a referral to another therapist for a second opinion.

When terminating therapy, you should give your clients as much notice as possible. Having therapy abruptly terminated is stressful for clients, particularly for those who have abandonment issues. Giving advance notice will give you and your clients time to prepare emotionally for the termination. Clients that you anticipate may particularly struggle with terminations may be informed even as early as 2–3 months in advance, if possible. This permits you to solicit and process your clients' fears regarding changing therapists. Advance notice of termination may also motivate your clients to work harder in therapy to avoid having to change therapists.

You also need to make sure that clients are properly transferred or referred if therapy should be continued. When making an outside referral, you should ideally provide your clients with two or more referrals so they have several choices. This increases the likelihood of finding a suitable therapist. If you are going to transfer your clients to another therapist within the agency or practice, then it's ideal if the two of you can have a conjoint session with the clients, which provides the most continuity for both the clients and the new therapist. The two of you may even do some type of intervention or ritual to formally symbolize the transfer of the clients from one therapist to another. For example, the new therapist may primarily take an observing role during the transfer session, but deliver a summarizing message at the end of the session to mark his or her greater involvement in the case from that point forward.

CLIENT TERMINATIONS

Unilateral terminations, whether initiated by the client or therapist, are usually frustrating for the party that was not consulted. What can make client terminations even more difficult is that they can occur without warning, and the client may never offer an explanation for terminating therapy. The client may simply not show up for therapy, or might cancel the appointment and never reschedule. Therapist reactions to client terminations include blaming the client ("They were unmotivated"), being relieved ("They were a difficult case"), acceptance ("This happens to all therapists, it is just part of doing therapy"), or blaming oneself ("I must have done something wrong").

Beginning therapists frequently worry when a client does not return to therapy that they have done something wrong. However, you should not automatically assume that a termination is a sign of failure on your part. This point was poignantly made for one of the authors (L. W.) during two internship cases. One couple who had suddenly dropped out of therapy came back unexpectedly after 5 months. When I expressed surprise at seeing them return, they explained how a number of events such as a job change and move had made it difficult to continue therapy. However, they expressed eagerness to continue with therapy because they had found our work together helpful.

A second couple came in approximately 2 weeks later, and reported that another couple had strongly recommended me based on their experience with me. I was surprised by the strong recommendation because the couple who had made the referral had dropped out of therapy unexpectedly.

Clients can terminate therapy for a variety of reasons. For some clients, the problem may simply be resolved and they no longer see the need to continue therapy. As in the preceding example, you may get referrals from these clients even though they terminated somewhat unexpectedly.

Other clients simply may lose momentum in coming to therapy. They may cancel an appointment (due to illness) or promise to call later to reschedule (after returning from vacation or a business trip). For these individuals, therapy may have helped to partially resolve the problem. The clients may have obtained enough relief that they no longer feel compelled to reinitiate or continue with therapy (Heath, 1988).

Some clients may discontinue therapy because they feel the costs of continuing it are too high. These costs can be financial, but they can also be costs in terms of emotional energy, time, and difficulty in getting to the therapist. For example, one single mother with three young children who came in for one session said she didn't return because she found an agency that provided home-based services.

Some clients will not return because they are dissatisfied with therapy. They may feel the therapist doesn't understand them or that change is not happening quickly enough. The dissatisfaction may be rooted in unrealistic expectations of what therapy is, or it may be because the therapist has been ineffective or has damaged the therapeutic relationship.

You should ideally follow up with clients who terminate without an explanation (Heath, 1988). Your next step will depend on the reason the client terminated therapy. You might be able to negotiate a lower fee for clients who terminate for financial reasons. If you have harmed the therapeutic relationship, you can attempt to fix the relationship, or at a minimum provide referrals for your clients. In some cases, you might want to invite your clients in for a termination session to bring a proper closure to therapy.

Terminations can be a difficult time for clients and therapists alike, particularly if termination is not mutually agreed upon by both parties. When the therapist must initiate termination, there is the potential for clients to feel abandoned or insecure about starting therapy with another therapist. Conversely, therapists may question whether they were effective in helping clients who appear to have prematurely left therapy. Even when terminating therapy is mutually agreed upon because goals for therapy have been successfully achieved, there can still be a sense of loss from ending the therapeutic relationship. An effective termination will deal with the losses and will also help clients consolidate the gains they have made and give them greater confidence about the future.

12

Family Therapy in the Future: Pertinent Issues for Beginning Clinicians

Beginning family therapists exit graduate school and enter the mental health marketplace with a noble goal—to help clients alleviate their distress and suffering. But in the therapist's office of the 21st century, the challenge of doing therapy will go beyond the "basics" encountered during training. Clinical work in many settings will mean cooperating and sharing turf with other health care providers, giving increased attention to individual and DSM-IV diagnoses, adhering to treatment guidelines provided by someone else, and complying with utilization reviews. More than ever, family therapists may find themselves playing double advocate roles: searching out creative options for clients whose health care plans limit modality and length of treatment, and helping the profession prove its legitimacy, thereby ensuring that family therapy is one department in the "supermarket" of managed care.

Managed care is the current leader in health care reform, a complicated and evolving business in which government, industry, and providers are finding new ways to limit skyrocketing health care costs. Whatever form the new "system" takes, family therapists can be certain the effects will be felt by themselves and their clients. Although there is tremendous variability by region in the prevalence of managed care, it is only a matter of time until the health maintenance organization (HMO), based on primary care, controls health care delivery (Jancin, 1993). In this chapter, we leave you with a glimpse of the present and future "business" of family therapy, the implications (pro and con) for your work with clients, and some pointers that will help you navigate the unpredictable waters of health care reform.

MANAGED CARE: IMPLICATIONS FOR YOU
AND YOUR CLIENTS

Managed competition may mean "good news" and "bad news" for consumers and providers of mental health services, and family therapists should be aware of both sides of the story. The good news is that a significant number of Americans who were previously uninsured will have access to care. Increasing access to care for these groups is a goal that resonates with the values of family therapists. We will be choosing among different health care plans which all offer basic services but may vary in others, including the emphasis on mental health care—a spectrum of plans ranging from catastrophic to comprehensive coverage will be available.

At the same time, clients may be "caught" in the managed care company's battle to balance cost-effectiveness with quality care. The practice of gatekeeping, for example, means that case managers and primary care physicians need to authorize referrals to and treatment by therapists. The potential here is for postponed treatment, bureaucratic obstacles that lead clients to give up, and severely limited choices regarding who the clients will see. In addition, numerous chronic problems and certain acute ones may not "qualify" for treatment. Similarly, time-limited therapy is the rule in managed care, despite the fact that resolution of some problems requires long-term treatment. Finally, in an environment where cost-effectiveness is so crucial, there may be an overreliance on drugs. The ease with which certain popular drugs are prescribed, and the use of these as diagnostic tools, may prevent clients from pursuing other types of treatment.

How managed care is "received" by family therapists depends on one's history. For some clinicians, especially those with a tradition of fee-for-service private practice, health care reform has created a foreboding of loss or fear; feeling squeezed out or taken over by managed care, they may struggle with loss of autonomy, control, reimbursement, and income. But for beginners, work in a managed care setting can mean a secure, steady income and a chance to join the crucial shift in health toward an interdisciplinary, biopsychosocial approach to wellness.

Indeed, master's-level family therapists may have an advantage in managed care organizations, as do master's-level nurse practitioners and certified physician assistants. Providing quality care for common problems in the least expensive way is fundamental to the new health care organization. Family therapists are likely to practice on a team with clinical psychologists, psychiatrists, and primary care physicians in order to address the health care needs of a population. The closer the family therapist is to the primary care physician, the better a biopsychosocial approach to health care can be maintained.

When the primary care physician and family therapist meet together around the care of a person and family, a greater efficiency of care will complement the quality of services. Since one primary care physician cares for 1,500–2,000 patients, there would be two primary care physicians for every mental health provider in a managed care setting. New models of integrating mental health providers with primary care physicians will be able to flourish under managed care since capitation—the practice of paying a set fee for the health care of particular populations—liberates the providers from having to worry about coding, charges, and reimbursement from a common office.

WHAT EVERY FAMILY THERAPIST NEEDS TO KNOW

Whatever the pros and cons of the current managed care environment, changes in how health care is provided and received are here to stay. While the "old days" may be over for veterans in family therapy, many new therapists (if not most) will begin their professional careers within organized care delivery systems. Issues of autonomy probably will not be foremost in the minds of beginning therapists, but becoming part of a managed care team will. The summary that follows provides new family therapists with the essentials to understand, prepare for, and navigate in a managed care environment.

1. *Managed care means an emphasis on primary care.* Primary care generally refers to the medical specialties of pediatrics, internal medicine, and family medicine. These primary care physicians will serve as case managers and be responsible for all facets of their patients' clinical care and resource management. Primary care-focused health care delivery is economical and relies less on technological treatments and more on education and prevention. A switch toward emphasizing primary care could be a positive change for family therapists because of the historical and philosophical links between family therapy and family medicine. Whether you work directly for a managed care company as an employee-provider, or provide services as an HMO panel member, maintaining a working relationship with physicians will be important.

2. *In general, reimbursement for services is going to move from a fee-for-service system to a capitated system.* Fee-for-service means a thera-

pist provides a professional service, for example, an hour of therapy, and gets paid for that service. Capitation refers to a therapist (or group of therapists) assuming responsibility for all mental health needs of a specific identified population and then being paid a set amount for assuming that responsibility, regardless of the frequency and intensity of services provided within a specific time frame.

The positive side of capitation is that the therapist need not withhold treatment because the family cannot afford therapy. The negative side is that some treatments deemed necessary by the therapist may still not be covered by the managed care plan, while others may be time-limited. Family therapists need to use authorized sessions creatively, perhaps using alternatives to the standard of the weekly, 50-minute hour.

Since capitation puts the burden of cost containment partially on the provider, family therapists must have some knowledge of case management and practice economics. Family therapists must be trained to think about issues regarding treatment efficiency, effectiveness, cost, patient satisfaction, utilization, and access.

3. *Comprehensive service delivery with the primary care physician as case manager is the goal of managed care.* Thus, family therapists must be able to work as part of an interdisciplinary team, which might include a primary care physician, a dietitian, a nurse practitioner, a psychiatrist, and any other health care specialist deemed necessary for effective treatment. Embedded in working as part of an interdisciplinary team are issues of loss of autonomy, establishing parity or hierarchical relationship with other health care providers, and credibility regarding the services provided by family therapy (compared to the more clearly measured outcomes of biological sciences and medical model treatments). Family therapists must understand how other specialists think about problems, for example, the psychiatrist's focus on individual physical symptoms or the family physician's focus on pragmatic, efficient treatment (Patterson & Magulac, 1994). The ability to actively consult with and understand other professionals while communicating the role of family therapy is essential.

4. *In managed care, a specific diagnosis and treatment plan will be important.* Because of utilization management, outcome research, and other macro accountability methods, a clear articulation of the problem, possible treatments, chosen treatment, and expected outcomes is critical. In other words, family therapists need to convey appropriate information to managed care companies and must be aware of specific criteria. For example, obtaining treatment authorization often includes the following: documenting a DSM-IV diagnosis, level of impaired functioning, level of care needed, and prognosis. Proving "medical necessity" means addressing both diagnostic and functional criteria. While Axis I diagnoses indi-

cate acuteness and medical need, the more chronic Axis II conditions may not be sufficient to obtain treatment authorization. Clinicians can focus on the acute manifestation of an Axis II disorder, which likely brought the client into therapy. In addition to providing a DSM-IV diagnosis, therapists may need to give evidence of clinical instability, which includes potential lethality to self or other, current medical status, and ability to perform basic self-care. In documenting authorizations, therapists will also address interpersonal relationships and a client's ability to maintain vocational and other activities—problems here might be classified as functional impairments.

While some diagnoses (e.g., phobias) have strict diagnostic criteria and convincing treatment outcome research, other issues frequently discussed in therapy are more vague or would not be covered by most managed care plans. For example, most plans would not cover marital therapy to treat communication problems. However, a distressed spouse might tell his primary care physician that he is depressed and is not eating or sleeping because of a painful marriage. Part of the treatment for depression might be marital therapy (Coyne, 1988). Whatever the identified problem and treatment goals, therapists need to use behavioral terms that reflect symptom reduction. Treatment modality also needs to be identified and rationalized. For family therapists, obtaining treatment authorization may mean a documented focus on the IP and his or her symptoms rather than on systemic or relational issues and etiologies.

5. Quality management will be an important part of managed care. This term refers to the basic systems, policies, and procedures providers must implement to assure improved outcomes and quality of service (Scherger, 1994). There are three major categories of quality management, according to Eidus and Warburton (1990): (a) structure—how the health care delivery system is organized; (b) process—how patients receive care; and (c) outcome—an objective measure of the health of an individual or population. These concepts are familiar to family therapists who have been taught to think structurally throughout their training and have been exposed to both process and outcome research on therapeutic effectiveness. Thus, it's a small step for family therapists to apply these issues in a practical way at a macro level in their clinical setting. Early family therapy initiatives in process and outcome research in HMO primary care are focusing on how therapy can affect utilization by patients with chronic pain, somatization, depression, and anxiety (Bloch, 1994).

In practical terms, family therapists need to identify and document the focus of treatment early, and use behavioral terms. They also need to be familiar with the utilization review practices of any managed care company with which they work. Progress notes must be legible and up-to-date, and should demonstrate some measure of change noted from session to session. Further, therapists need to show reviewers that applicable treatment guidelines or current standards for treatment are being followed.

6. *Resource management skills will be necessary for the family therapist working within an HMO.* The relationship between continued therapy and patient improvement is an important consideration. Group therapies that prove as effective as individual therapies may take precedence in managed care because they are cost effective. Since family therapists have been working with family groups and systems, they should already have the necessary skills to make this transition.

Solution-focused therapists and psychoeducational family therapists have articulated treatment goals that are narrower in focus and less ambitious than cure. Minimal intervention necessary for improvement and stabilizing or improving the family's situation are frequent goals of these therapies. Indeed, many clinical treatments have a ceiling effect: that is, the situation improves to a certain degree, and after that ceiling is reached, continued treatment and resource investment will produce few and negligible gains.

7. *Finally, patient satisfaction is very important, and measured, in managed care, so therapists must know their patients.* This should be an area where family therapists excel, since relationship skills have always been a basic ingredient of family therapy. Research suggests that patients' most frequent complaints and reasons for changing doctors include (a) the physician doesn't care, (b) the physician doesn't listen, or (c) the physician doesn't explain in a way that is understandable (Desmond, 1993). The right to choose one's personal physician has been a contentious issue in the current health care debate and reflects patients' concerns about choosing, knowing, and being cared for by their physician (and therapist).

Training clinics routinely incorporate patient satisfaction measures into their protocol, but this process can be overlooked in a time-consuming private practice. Managed care presents the opportunity of obtaining macro measures of patient satisfaction and feedback for the family therapist who wants to know how to improve clinical services.

In the past, the family therapist's focus was on helping families function more effectively, usually by altering their interactions. Today, new family therapists must also think about cost-effectiveness, research effectiveness versus the practical efficacy of using a treatment in the "real world," criteria for treatment authorization, treatment guidelines, time-limited therapies, utilization reviews, accountability. The approach may be interdisciplinary and biopsychosocial, and family therapists will become team members who share with other professionals a concern for the client's total health. By expanding beyond the boundaries of traditional family therapy training and gaining understanding of the forces shaping health care services, beginning family therapists can help themselves and their clients maximize the benefits and minimize the detrimental aspects of managed care.

THE QUESTION THAT BINDS: WHAT HARMS AND WHAT HELPS?

In many ways, health care reform and managed care are demanding that the profession of family therapy be accountable and demonstrate real value. The question that drives the business of psychotherapy—with its focus on cost-effectiveness and client satisfaction—is relevant to beginning therapists not simply because they may find themselves answering to utilization review boards, but because this most basic of issues has a personal, as well as financial, bearing on the work we do.

As managed care companies develop treatment guidelines for specific psychological problems, they ask an underlying question which research attempts to answer: "Does this treatment alleviate this problem?" Likewise, beginning therapists often find themselves asking, "Is therapy really helping my clients?" Frequently, the question is posed during moments of angst or disillusionment, when clients drop out of treatment, backslide, or in some way show us that, despite our efforts and theirs, therapy is not "succeeding."

The question of what helps or hurts in psychotherapy, and to what degree, is valid across so many domains of the profession and so fundamental to future therapists that we devote our final discussion in this book to it.

Consumer Reports (1995) raised the question "Does therapy help?" An equally provocative questions is "Does therapy harm clients?" Research on both questions from the client's and therapist's perspectives demonstrate that both outcomes are possible.

The *Consumer Reports* article surveyed consumers of therapy and found the following:

1. In general, the discipline of the therapist didn't matter in terms of client satisfaction with therapy (unfortunately, the study did not distinguish between marriage counselors and licensed or certified marriage and family therapists).
2. Consumers who saw their family doctor for a mental health problem improved but those who saw a mental health specialist for more than 6 months did even better.
3. The longer people stayed in therapy, the more they felt they improved.

4. Consumers of group therapies were very satisfied, especially those who were members of Alcoholics Anonymous.

The article suggests that this consumer-oriented self-report study more accurately reflects "real world" problems than the experimental design with its use of control groups in measuring effectiveness of psychotherapy. Reflecting the consumers' enthusiasm for psychotherapy, the article concludes that "therapy works!"

Consumer enthusiasm for psychotherapy is in marked contrast to the psychotherapy field's more critical evaluation. Neil Jacobson and Alan Gurman (1995) differentiate between statistical and clinical significance when looking at therapeutic outcome. They state that, "when psychotherapy outcome is examined under the microscope of clinical significance, its effect appears to be quite modest, even for disorders that are thought to be easily treated" (p. 43).

Jacobson (1995) summarizes the results of the largest outcome study ever done on depression by saying, "Thus only a minority of patients recovered and stayed recovered for more than a year. Even the placebo treatment did as well. Neither pharmacotherapy nor psychotherapy led to lasting recovery for the great majority of cases" (p. 46). Allen Bergin (1991) conducted a meta-analysis of outcome studies in the 1960s and argued that 5–10% of clients even got worse during therapy.

Perhaps other variables can explain the effectiveness or failure of psychotherapy. Jacobson states that there is overwhelming evidence that psychotherapy outcome is not improved either by years of clinical experience or by professional training. While there is evidence that some therapies work better for some problems than others, in general the theoretical orientation used in therapy does not strongly influence outcome.

What factors do explain outcome? Research suggests that the most powerful predictors of a positive therapy outcome are qualities the client brings to therapy—motivation, beliefs that therapy will help, confidence and trust in the therapist, and history. Beyond the client's qualities, the therapeutic relationship appears to be the other important predictor, as Grunebaum (1988) points out: "Mainly what goes on between the patient and the therapist is what matters . . . and what matters the most about the therapeutic bond is what the [clients] think it is like" (p. 197).

While therapist–client interaction can greatly help clients, it is equally plausible that clients can be harmed. Factors that harm clients include (1) confronting clients defenses too quickly; (2) a therapist who is cold, aloof, or distant; (3) inappropriate boundaries between client and therapist; and (4) rigid adherence to one theory (Grunebaum, 1988). Encouraging clients to express socially unacceptable feelings such as rage or sexual feelings and then criticizing them for those feelings can be harmful as well.

Another factor that can harm clients is lack of access to treatment. People with mental disorders have a diminished quality of life. Future therapists who want to help their clients will face dilemmas unknown in earlier years. They may have clients whose health plan doesn't pay for mental health treatments or only pays for a limited number of sessions. In addition to developing strong therapeutic relationship skills, therapists in training must become advocates for their clients, helping them to get the services they need.

Student therapists can recognize that while their program may emphasize learning theory and technique, and while managed care's emphasis on mental health may mean writing behavioral treatment objectives, having measurable goals, and utilizing concise treatment plans following a review committee's guidelines, these skills have very little to do with therapeutic outcome. Instead, it's the softer, more difficult-to-measure qualities that will determine a therapist's effectiveness: Does the therapist care about his or her client? Is the therapist competent and able to motivate a client? Can the therapist communicate hope and warmth? These elusive qualities will largely determine your success as a therapist, while research continues to pave the way for the future of family therapy.

References

Ahrons, C. (1994). *The good divorce.* New York: HarperCollins.

Ahrons, C. R., & Rodgers, R. H. (1987). *Divorced families: A multidisciplinary view.* New York: Norton.

Alexander, J., Holtzworth-Munroe, A., & Jameson, P. (1994). The process and outcome of marital and family therapy: Research review and evaluation. In A. Bergin & A. Garfield (Eds.), *Handbook of psychotherapy and behavior change* (pp. 595–630). New York: Wiley.

American heritage dictionary, The. (2nd college ed.). (1985). Boston: Houghton Mifflin.

American Psychiatric Association. (1994). *Diagnostic and statistical manual of mental disorders* (4th ed.). Washington, DC: Author.

Anderson, C. M., & Stewart, S. (1983). *Mastering resistance: A practical guide to family therapy.* New York: Guilford Press.

Aponte, H. (1976). Underorganization in the poor family. In P. J. Guerin (Ed.), *Family therapy: Theory and practice.* New York: Gardner Press.

Barlow, D. H. (Ed.). (1993). *Clinical handbook of psychological disorders: A step-by-step treatment manual* (2nd ed.). New York: Guilford Press.

Berger, D., & Berger, L., (1991). *We heard the angels of madness.* New York: Morrow.

Bergin, A. (1991). Values and religious issues in psychotherapy and mental health. *American Psychologist, 46*(4), 394–403.

Bergin, A., & Garfield, S. (Eds.). (1994). *Handbook of psychotherapy and behavior change* (4th ed.). New York: Wiley.

Berrill, K. T. (1990). Anti-gay violence and victimization in the United States: An overview. *Journal of Interpersonal Violence, 5,* 274–294.

Bloch, D. (1994, January). *Collaborative family health care.* Paper presented at the Collaborative Family Health Care: Opportunities and Directions, Racine, WI.

Brown, E. M. (1991). *Patterns of infidelity and their treatment.* New York: Brunner/Mazel.

235

Buck, J., & Jolles, I. (1966). *House-Tree-Person*. Los Angeles: Western Psychological Services.

Bureau of National Affairs, Inc. (1982). *The Uniform Marriage and Divorce Act.* Section 402.

Carter, B., & McGoldrick, M. (1989). *The changing family life cycle*. Boston: Allyn & Bacon.

Clarkin, J. F., & Glick, I. (1992). *A manual for psychoeducational marital intervention of bipolar disorder*. New York: Cornell Medical Center.

Clarkin, J. F., Haas, G. L., & Glick, I. D. (Eds.). (1988). *Affective disorders and the family*. New York: Guilford Press.

Colon, F. (1980). Overview: The changing family life cycle. In E. A. Carter & M. McGoldrick (Eds.), *The family life cycle: A framework for family therapy* (p. 15). New York: Gardner Press.

Connell, J. (1995, December 6). Bridging gap between faith and medicine. *San Diego Union–Tribune*, p. D-1.

Connors, C. K. (1987). *Connors rating scale revised technical manual*. New York: MultiHealth Systems.

Consumer Reports. (1995). Mental health: Does therapy help? *11*, 734–739.

Coyne, J. (1988). Strategic therapy. In J. F. Clarkin, G. L. Haas, & I. D. Glick (Eds.), *Affective disorders and the family* (pp. 89–113). New York: Guilford Press.

Crane, D., Newfield, N., & Armstrong, D. (1984). Predicting divorce at marital therapy intake: Wives' distress and the marital status inventory. *Journal of Marital and Family Therapy, 10*(3), 305–312.

Craske, M., & Zoellner, L. (1995). Anxiety disorders: The role of marital therapy. In N. S. Jacobson & A. S. Gurman (Eds.), *Clinical handbook of couple therapy* (pp. 394–410). New York: Guilford Press.

Dadds, M. (1995). *Families, children and the development of dysfunction*. Thousands Oaks, CA: Sage.

Davenport, Y. B., & Adland, M. L. (1988). Management of manic episodes. In J. F. Clarkin, G. L. Haas, & I. D. Glick (Eds.), *Affective disorders and the family* (pp. 173–195). New York: Guilford Press.

Denton, W. (1990). A family systems analysis of DSM-III-R. *Journal of Marital and Family Therapy, 16*(2), 113–125.

Denton, W., Patterson, J., & Van Meir, E. (1997). Use of the DSM in marriage and family therapy programs: Current practices and attitudes. *Journal of Marital and Family Therapy, 23*(1), 81–86.

Desmond, J. (1993, October). *The physician–patient relationship*. Paper presented at the meeting Managed Care: An Approach for the Physician, San Diego County Medical Society, San Diego, CA.

Dilsaver, S. C. (1990). The mental status examination. *American Family Physician, 41*(5), 1489–1497.

Doherty, W., & Simmons, D. (1995). Defining who we are and what we do: Clinical practice patterns of marriage and family therapists in Minnesota. *Journal of Marriage and Family Therapy, 21*(1), 3–16.

Duvall, E. (1955). *Family development*. New York: Lippincott.

Edwards, D. L., & Gil, E. (1986). *Breaking the cycle: Assessment and treatment of child abuse and neglect.* Los Angeles: Association for Advanced Training in the Behavioral Sciences.

Edwards, J., Johnson, D., & Booth, A. (1987). Coming apart: A prognostic instrument of marital breakup. *Journal of Applied Family and Child Studies, 36*(2), 168–170.

Edwards, M., & Steinglass, P. (1995). Family therapy treatment outcomes for alcoholism. *Journal of Marital and Family Therapy, 21*(4), 475–509.

Eidus, R., & Warburton, S. (1990). *Managed care: A teaching syllabus.* Kansas City, MO: Society of Teachers of Family Medicine.

Estrada, A., & Pinsof, W. (1995). The effectiveness of family therapies for selected behavioral disorders of childhood. *Journal of Marital and Family Therapy, 4,* 403–440.

Ewing, J. A. (1984). Detecting alcoholism: The CAGE questionnaire. *Journal of the American Medical Association, 252,* 1905–1907.

Figley, C. R., & Nelson, T. S. (1989). Basic family therapy skills, I: Conceptualization and initial findings. *Journal of Marital and Family Therapy, 15*(4), 349–365.

Finkelhor, D., Hotaling, G., Lewis, I. A., & Smith, C. (1990). Sexual abuse in a national survey of adult men and women: Prevalence, characteristics and risk-factors. *Child Abuse, 14,* 19–28.

Finley, G. (1997). *Intimate enemy: Winning the war within yourself.* St. Paul, MN: Llewellyn.

Fisch, R., Weakland, J. H., & Segal, L. (1985). *The tactics of change: Doing therapy briefly.* San Francisco: Jossey-Bass.

Fitchett, G. (1993). *Spiritual assessment in pastoral care: A guide to selected resources.* Decatur, GA: Journal of Pastoral Care Publications.

Fournier, D. G., Olson, D. H., & Druckman, J. M. (1983). Assessing marital and premarital relationships: The prepare/enrich inventories. In E. E. Filsinger (Ed.), *Marriage and family assessment* (pp. 229–250). Newbury Park, CA: Sage.

Garbarino, J., & Stott, F. (1989). *What children can tell us: Eliciting, interpreting, and evaluating information from children.* San Francisco: Jossey-Bass.

Goering, P., & Rhodes, A. (1994). Gender differences in the use of outpatient mental health services. *Journal of Mental Health Administration, 21*(4), 338–346.

Goldner, V. (1985). Feminism and family therapy. *Family Process, 24,* 31–47.

Gordon, M., & Creighton, S. J. (1988). Natal and non-natal fathers as sexual abusers in the United Kingdom: A comparative analysis. *Journal of Marriage and the Family, 50,* 99–105.

Gotlib, I., & Beach, S. (1995). A marital/family discord model of depression: Implications for therapeutic intervention. In N. S. Jacobson & A. S. Gurman (Eds.), *Clinical handbook of couple therapy* (pp. 411–436). New York: Guilford Press.

Gottman, J. M. (1994). *What predicts divorce?* Hillsdale, NJ: Erlbaum.

Greenberg, L. S., & Johnson, S. M. (1988). *Emotionally focused therapy for couples.* New York: Guilford Press.

Griffith, J. L., & Griffith, M. E. (1994). *The body speaks: Therapeutic dialogues for mind–body problems.* New York: Basic Books.

Grunebaum, H. (1988). What if family therapy were a kind of psychotherapy?: A reading of the handbook of psychology and behavioral change. *Journal of Marital and Family Therapy, 14*(2), 195–199.

Gurman, A. S., & Kniskern, D. P. (Eds.). (1991). *Handbook of family therapy.* New York: Brunner/Mazel.

Heath, A. W. (1988). Ending family therapy: Some new directions. *Family Therapy Collections, 14,* 33–40.

Hirschfeld, R., & Russell, J. (1997). Assessment and treatment of suicidal patients. *New England Journal of Medicine, 337*(13), 910–915.

Hoffman, L. (1981). *Foundations of family therapy.* New York: Basic Books.

Imber-Black, E. (1988). *Families and larger systems: A family therapist's guide through the labyrinth.* New York: Guilford Press.

Jacobson, N. S., & Gurman, A. S. (Eds.). (1995). *Clinical handbook of couple therapy.* New York: Guilford Press.

James, K., & McIntyre, D. (1983). The reproduction of families: The social role of the family. *Journal of Marital and Family Therapy, 9,* 119–129.

Jancin, B. (1993). Why the future of health care might "look a lot like San Diego." *Family Practice News, 11,* 38.

Jongsma, A. E., & Peterson, L. M. (1996). *The complete psychotherapy treatment planner.* New York: Wiley.

Keitner, G., Ryan, C., Miller, I., & Kohn, R. (1993). The role of the family in major depressive illness. *Psychiatric Annals, 23*(9), 500–507.

Kessler, R., Eaton, W., Wittchen, H., & Zhao, S. (1994). DSM-III-R: Generalized anxiety disorder in the national comorbidity survey. *Archives of General Psychiatry, 51*(5), 355–364.

Kilpatrick, A. C. (1987). Childhood sexual experiences: Problems and issues in studying long-range effects. *Journal of Sex Research, 22,* 221–242.

Kitchens, J. M. (1994). Does this patient have an alcohol problem? *Journal of the American Medical Association, 272*(22), 1782–1787.

Lauer, J. W., Lourie, I. S., Salus, M. K., & Broadhurst, D. D. (1979). *The role of the mental health professional in the prevention and treatment of child abuse and neglect.* Washington, DC: U.S. Department of Health, Education, Welfare, National Center on Child Abuse and Neglect.

Leber, D., St. Peters, M., & Markman, H. J. (1996). Program evaluation research: Applications to marital and family therapy. In D. H. Sprenkle & S. M. Moon (Eds.), *Research methods in family therapy* (pp. 485–506). New York: Guilford Press.

Liddle, H., & Dakof, G. (1995). Efficacy of family therapy for drug abuse: Promising but not definitive. *Journal of Marital and Family Therapy, 21*(4), 511–543.

Lindblad-Goldberg, M. (1989). Successful minority single-parent families. In L. Combrinck-Graham (Ed.), *Children in family contexts* (pp. 116–134). New York: Guilford Press.

Locke, H. J., & Wallace, K. M. (1959). Short term marital adjustment and prediction tests: Their reliability and validity. *Journal of Marriage and Family Living, 21,* 251–255.

Markman, H. J. (1987). *The prediction and prevention of marital distress* (Annual report). Rockville, MD: National Institute of Mental Health.

McCollum, E. E. (1990). Integrating structural–strategic and Bowen approaches in training beginning family therapists. *Contemporary Family Therapy, 12,* 23–34.

McCrady, B., & Epstein, E., (1995). Marital therapy in the treatment of alcohol problems. In N. S. Jacobson & A. S. Gurman (Eds.), *Clinical handbook of couple therapy* (pp. 369–393). New York: Guilford Press.

McGoldrick, M., & Gerson, R. (1985). *Genograms in family assessment.* New York: Norton.

McGrath, E., Keita, G. P., Strickland, B. R., & Russon, N. F. (1990). *Woman and depression: Risk factors and treatment issues.* Washington, DC: American Psychological Association.

McGuire, L., & Wagner, N. (1978). Sexual dysfunction in women who were molested as children. *Sex and Marriage, 4,* 11–15.

The Medical Letter. (1991). *The medical letter on drugs and therapeutics, 33*(844), 43–50.

Miklowitz, D. J., & Goldstein, M. J. (1997). *Bipolar disorder: A family-focused treatment approach.* New York: Guilford Press.

Minuchin, S., & Fishman, H. C. (1981). *Family therapy techniques.* Cambridge, MA: Harvard University Press.

Minuchin, S., Montalvo, B., Guerney, B. G., Rosman B. L., & Schumer, F. (1967). *Families of the slums.* New York: Basic Books.

Moltz, D. (1993). Bipolar disorder and the family: An integrative model. *Family Process, 32*(4), 409–423.

Nichols, M. P., & Schwartz, R. C. (1991). *Family therapy: Concepts and methods.* Boston: Allyn & Bacon.

Nichols, W. C. (1988). *Marital therapy: An integrative approach.* New York: Guilford Press.

O'Brian, C., & Bruggen, P. (1985). Our personal and professional lives: Learning positive connotation and circular questions. *Family Process, 24,* 311–322.

O'Hanlon, W. (1982). Strategic pattern intervention. *Journal of Strategic and Systemic Therapies, 4,* 26–33.

Patterson, G. R. (1990). *Depression and aggression in family interactions.* Hillsdale, NJ: Erlbaum.

Patterson, J. E., & Magulac, M. (1994). The family therapist's guide to psychopharmacology: A graduate level course. *Journal of Marital and Family Therapy, 20*(2), 151–173.

Piercy, F., & Sprenkle, P. (1990). Marriage and family therapy: A decade review. *Journal of Marriage and the Family, 52,* 1116–1126.

Pittman, F. S. (1987). *Turning points: Treating families in transition and crisis.* New York: Norton.

Pfeiffer, E. (1975). A short portable mental status questionnaire for the assessment of organic brain deficit in elderly patients. *Journal of the American Geriatric Society, 23,* 433–441.

Prince, S., & Jacobson, N. (1995). Couple and family therapy for depression. In

E. E. Beckham & W. R. Leber (Eds.), *Handbook of depression* (2nd ed., pp. 404–424). New York: Guilford Press.

Rappaport, L. (1970). Crisis intervention as a brief mode of treatment. In R. W. Roberts & R. H. Nee (Eds.), *Theories of social casework* (pp. 123–159). Chicago: University of Chicago Press.

Rogers, C. R. (1972). *On becoming a person.* Boston: Houghton Mifflin.

Rubin, L. (1983). *Intimate strangers.* New York: HarperCollins.

Sanderson, W. C. (1995). Can psychological interventions meet the new demands of health care? *American Journal of Managed Care, 1*(1), 93–98.

Satir, V. (1967). *Conjoint family therapy.* Palo Alto, CA: Science & Behavior Books.

Saunders, J. B., Aasland, O. G., Babor, T. F., De La Fuente, J. R., & Grant, M. (1993). Development of the Alcohol Use Disorders Identification Test: WHO Collaborative project on early detection of persons with harmful alcohol consumption II. *Addiction, 88,* 791–804.

Scherger, J. (1994). Does managed care contaminate practice? *Family Practice Management, 1,* 94–100.

Selzer, M. L. (1971). The Michigan Alcoholism Screening Test: The quest for a new diagnostic instrument. *American Journal of Psychiatry, 127,* 1653–1658.

Shea, M. T., Gibbons, R., Elkin, I., & Sotsky, S. (1995). Initial severity and differential treatment outcome in the National Institute of Mental Health treatment of depression of collaborative research program. *Journal of Consulting and Clinical Psychology, 63*(5), 841–847.

Shields, C., Wynne, L. C., McDaniel, S. H., & Gawuisler, B. A. (1994). The marginalization of family therapy: A historical and continuing problem. *Journal of Marital and Family Therapy, 20*(1), 117–138.

Snyder, D. K. (1979). Multidimensional assessment of marital satisfaction. *Journal of Marriage and the Family, 41*(4), 813–823.

Spanier, G. B. (1976). Measuring marital adjustment: New scales for assessing the quality of marriage and similar dyads. *Journal of Marriage and Family, 38,* 15–28.

Sprenkle, D. H., & Bischoff, R. J. (1991). Research in family therapy: Trends, issues and recommendations. In M. Nichols & R. Schwartz (Eds.), *Family therapy: Concepts and methods* (pp. 542–580). Boston: Allyn & Bacon.

Steinglass, P., Bennett, L. A., Wolin, S. J., & Reiss. D. (1987). *The alcoholic family.* New York: Basic Books.

Sue, D. W., & Sue, D. (1980). *Counseling the culturally different: Theory and practice.* New York: Wiley.

Taggart, M. (1985). The feminist critique in epistemological perspective: Questions of context in family therapy. *Journal of Marital and Family Therapy, 11,* 113–126.

Tannen, D. (1990). *You just don't understand: Men and women in conversation.* New York: Ballantine.

Taylor, R. (1990). *Distinguishing psychological from organic disorders: Screening for psychological masquerades.* New York: Springer.

Thorman, G. (1980). *Family violence.* Springfield, IL: Charles C Thomas.

Tomm, K. (1988). Interventive interviewing: Part III. *Family Process, 27*(1), 1–15.

U.S. Department of Health and Human Services. (1993). *Depression in primary care: Clinical practice guidelines* (No. 5). Rockville, MD: Agency for Health Care and Policy and Research.

Walker, L. E. (1979). *The battered woman.* New York: Harper & Row.

Walker, L. E., & Hooper, A. (1982). *Management of the physically and emotionally abused.* Norwalk, CT: Appleton–Century–Crofts.

Wechsler, D. (1991). *Wechsler Intelligence Scale for Children* (3rd. ed.). San Antonio, TX: Psychological Corporation.

Weiss, R., & Cerrato, M. (1980). The marital status inventory: Development of a measure of dissolution potential. *American Journal of Family Therapy, 8*(2), 80–85.

Wolf, E. S. (1988). *Treating the self: Elements of clinical self psychology.* New York: Guilford Press.

Index